ADVANCE PRAISE FOR

Serving Refugee Children: Listening to Stories of Detention in the USA

"For reasons both ethical and bureaucratic, child migrants rarely tell their own stories. Yet the world needs to hear them if we are to find a way to end their suffering. In this valuable collection of reflections by activists and scholars, the reader begins to hear children's voices, to understand the lives of their caregivers, and to gain the possibility to stand with them in solidarity."

—Donna R. Gabaccia, Professor Emerita, University of Toronto

"*Serving Refugee Children* is timely and it's essential. The historical context provided by the introduction is a fact often neglected when trying to understand the desperate act of leaving everything behind in search of—not a better life but often, simply—a life.

The narratives of service providers that have come out of their experience caring for detained youth are an invaluable historical record and everlasting testimony. They reveal the human cost of policies fashioned by ideologues blinded by their own prejudices. The simple act of listening to the stories of these children dignifies their saga and is, in itself, an act of social justice."

—Luis Argueta, Director of the Documentary Series
abUSEd: The Postville Raid, ABRAZOS, and *The U Turn*

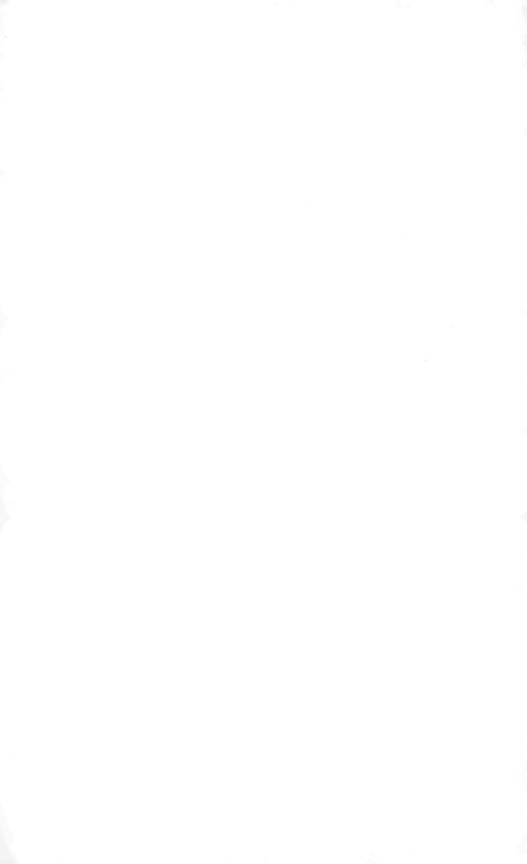

Serving Refugee Children

This book is part of the Peter Lang Regional Studies list.
Every volume is peer reviewed and meets
the highest quality standards for content and production.

PETER LANG

New York • Bern • Berlin
Brussels • Vienna • Oxford • Warsaw

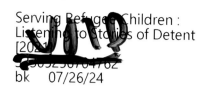

Serving Refugee Children

Listening to Stories of Detention in the USA

Edited by
Montse Feu and Amanda Venta

PETER LANG
New York • Bern • Berlin
Brussels • Vienna • Oxford • Warsaw

Library of Congress Cataloging-in-Publication Control Number: 2021016328

Bibliographic information published by **Die Deutsche Nationalbibliothek**.
Die Deutsche Nationalbibliothek lists this publication in the "Deutsche
Nationalbibliografie"; detailed bibliographic data are available
on the Internet at http://dnb.d-nb.de/.

ISBN 978-1-4331-7948-8 (hardcover)
ISBN 978-1-4331-7949-5 (paperback)
ISBN 978-1-4331-7950-1 (ebook pdf)
ISBN 978-1-4331-7951-8 (epub)
DOI 10.3726/b16756

© 2021 Peter Lang Publishing, Inc., New York
80 Broad Street, 5th floor, New York, NY 10004
www.peterlang.com

We hope the best for refugee children and hope they heal.
To those who serve and care.

CONTENTS

PREFACE

People in the United States (U.S.) and the world are outraged at the news of the separation of families and the detention of unaccompanied immigrant children at the U.S. border with Mexico. Since 2018, haunting news of children locked in cages and heartbreaking footage of children dying in immigration detention have alarmed the general public. On March 6, 2019, Representative Lauren Underwood reported the potential physical and psychological effects of separating migrant families and children at the border to the House Homeland Security Committee Secretary Kirstjen Nielsen.[1] Her report followed the leak of a memo that revealed U.S. government plans to forcibly separate migrant children from their families and deport them more quickly.[2] On July 2019, demonstrations started in front of several detention centers and in several U.S. cities with the campaign call "Never Again." After her visit to a detention facility, Member of Congress Alexandria Ocasio-Cortez denounced "a culture of cruelty" and a lack of accountability for inhumane practices in immigration detention.[3]

Similarly, reports and articles published in 2019 denounced conditions in immigrant detention centers as, "cruel, inhuman or degrading treatment that is prohibited by international law."[4] Cultural institutions, civic organizations, and politicians remain concerned about the humanitarian crisis at the border. In an effort to preserve artifacts that document this crisis, the Smithsonian drew international attention when it requested drawings by children that depict their living conditions in immigration detention.[5] Legally, two judges, one in California and one in the District of Columbia blocked former President Trump's asylum bans and restrictions. These legal, cultural, and political efforts have fought for humane border legislation and practices that are accountable to U.S. and international law.

However, the zero-tolerance policy implemented by the Trump Administration created a new form of unaccompanied children by separating families seeking refuge in the U.S. and created a pressing need for efforts drawing attention to families' experiences in incarceration. The humanitarian concerns about recent administrative decisions are enormous: migrant parents who crossed the border with their children were forcibly separated while they awaited criminal prosecution; even more troublesome, non-profit organizations have documented a number of parents being deported without their children. For instance, Texas Civil Rights Projects counted 2,000 children in U.S. custody who were separated from their family members as a result of this policy. *Serving Refugee Children: Listening to Stories of Detention in the USA* (henceforth, *Serving Refugee Children*) focuses mainly on the surge of children and adolescents migrating—many of them without any legal or even informal guardian—from Central America to the U.S. escaping regional violence, abuse, and deprivation in recent years.

Serving Refugee Children captures the experiences and sentiments of Central American undocumented and unaccompanied minors (up to 18-years-old) in immigration detention centers, immigration facilities, and schools from the perspective of the individuals who have served them and their families in recent years (2016 to present). This bilingual anthology grew from conversations with students at Sam Houston State University about their experiences working with refugee children. The manuscript aims to create a culture of empathy and justice for those who seek refuge by disseminating the stories heard by service providers who care for youth and families in detention. Identifying details in accounts have been modified for legal reasons. Nonetheless, their accounts reveal the unseemly treatment that refugee minors suffer today. Ultimately, *Serving Refugee Children* demands the abolishment of U.S. immigration detention as it is conceived today and calls for a move towards models of safety, support, and prevention.

Notes

1. Representative Lauren Underwood Facebook page, March 6, 2019. https://www.facebook.com/repunderwood/videos/2338476183098128/

2. Robert Crown Law Library Blog. Stanford Law School. http://liblog.law.stanford.edu/2019/01/memorandum-reveals-united-states-government-planned-to-traumatize-migrant-children/?fbclid=IwAR0SwaJtunt61twlm2OhWCxPJUG30gGQ5WvN8VAvt3YnRY-4GGdhJcvK41yA

3. "Reporting Exposes Border Patrol 'Culture of Cruelty'." Morning Joe. MSNBC, July 2, 2019.

4. Kennicott, Philip, "Will Our Migrant Detention Cages Be Studied in Tomorrow's Museums," *The Washington Post*, July 18, 2019.

5. Cohen, Elizabeth, and John Bonifield. "Smithsonian Interested in Obtaining Migrant Children's Drawings Depicting their Time in US Custody," *CNN*, July 8, 2019.

ACKNOWLEDGMENTS

Editors thank scholars and writers for their feedback in the drafts of this anthology: Chris Castañeda, Amelia Cotter, Donna R. Gabaccia, M. Miranda Maloney, Annelise Orleck, April Shemak, as well as the blind reviewers. They provided invaluable critical improvements to the collection. Editors also would like to thank Raquel Chiquillo, Wendy Herrera, Cristina Nava Wilson, and Jenny Patlan for assisting us in the revision of Spanish variations. Montse Feu also thanks students in her Spanish and Honors classes that discussed some of the stories of this collection.

INTRODUCTION: SERVING REFUGEE CHILDREN AND THEIR FAMILIES

Montse Feu and Amanda Venta

Serving Refugee Children started with Lupe,[1] a teacher in an immigration detention center in Texas, and her relationship with Luis, an unaccompanied child detained there. For 2 years she served as his teacher in the detention center. She was then asked to fly with him to the home of a distant relative, who would take custody of the child. Lupe did her best to keep Luis strong during his time in detention with reassuring words and expressions of care. Comforting the sad child was not easy—the rules of detention centers forbid touching or holding children, even when they are quite young. Concerned about the wellbeing of unaccompanied minors, Lupe's Associate professor of Hispanic Studies, Dr. Montse Feu, contacted Dr. Amanda Venta, Associate professor of Psychology, who had been providing psychological services for detained immigrant children since 2012. This edited volume was envisioned as a way to make known to the general public the ordeal that children like Luis endure. Contributors, Cassandra Bailey, Maria Baños Jordan, Melissa Briones, Yessica Colin, Amelia Cotter, Ana Maria Fores Tamayo, Luz M. Garcini, Estrella Godinez, Martin La Roche, Alfonso Mercado, Seth Michelson, Abigail Nunez-Saenz, Paola Quijano, Jaime Retamales, Juan Ríos Vega, Andy Torres, and Paloma and Francisco Villegas share the same principled commitment to advocating for the minors' wellbeing as Lupe, Montse, and Amanda. By foregrounding their valuable perspectives, *Serving Refugee Children* is committed to the reform and abolition of practices that compromise social justice and human rights.

In presenting the accounts written by those who serve children, *Serving Refugee Children* provides unprecedented access to one of the burning moral issues of our time. Contributing authors are volunteers or service providers in detention services and schools. They give a panoramic and grassroots view of their experience in serving refuge-seeking children. Contributing authors have spent many hours and sometimes years teaching, listening, and supporting the children and youth represented in these stories: Luz, Ximena, Toñito, Camila, Danny Mateo, Jeremías, Luis, Juan, Sheila, William, and Carlos.

The editors feel that sharing the experiences of these providers is a compelling political act of resistance to injustice and a call for action when legal constraints do not allow for the children's first-person narratives to be disclosed to the general public and the communities directly affected by these detention policies. Storytelling provides a close and intimate view of the emotional wounds and costs of child detention. Authors, in sharing children's strength and courage, demonstrate that justice, strength, compassion, and human connection are necessary for the wellbeing of refugee children.

The authorship of this anthology is indeed unique—rarely are the experiences activists, grassroots representatives, health and human services professionals, workers, researchers, teachers, and volunteers who serve unaccompanied minors in detention centers and schools disseminated to the general public. Authors Michelson, Fores Tamayo, and Baños Jordan volunteered providing poetry workshops in Spanish; Bailey, Colin and Godinez interviewed unaccompanied immigrant youth in centers and schools in Spanish with the goal of providing psychological services; Briones, Garcini and Laroche volunteer in respite and hospice centers; Lupe and Retamales worked and volunteered in detention centers; and the Villegas siblings and Ríos Vega have experienced discrimination in schools both in their own skin and in the stories of their students. The stories shared here show that authors soon become friends and allies that try to comfort unaccompanied minors. Readers will find fleeting moments of happiness, like when Toñito speaks his variety of Spanish with volunteers at the respite center that welcomes him, and finds joy playing with other children there. However, other stories demonstrate the lack of socialization and comforting physical interaction that children experience in detention and how this lack can cognitively and emotionally affect them.[2] By offering unprecedented access to children's experiences during or shortly after their detention in the U.S., the accounts in this volume ask readers to be concerned about refugee-seeking children and care for them.

On Storytelling

Although *Serving Refugee Children* is based on true events, names and identifying details of the unaccompanied minors have been changed to protect them. Storytelling and anonymity present a unique contribution of this anthology. Existing publications are limited in scope because, in providing identifying details about the youth involved, they require permission from both the child and the legal guardian prior to publication. This requirement produces two important selection biases. First, few stories are shared due to the difficulty of attaining these permissions. Second, only children who have a legal guardian available and willing to provide permission are represented in the available literature. This bias is particularly damaging given the current immigration context of the U.S., where a large number of children currently arriving to (or having recently arrived to) the U.S. come by themselves or are separated from their guardians at the U.S. border. Silencing these stories because of the impossibility of obtaining permission to publish is a tremendous disservice to the immigrant population. Relatedly, children who have come with or have been reunited with guardians in the U.S. are often in the care of an undocumented person. It is well documented that these adults readily fear deportation and avoid even much needed medical services due to fear of identifying themselves and the children under their care. Requiring the written permission of these caregivers therefore excludes the very families who are most marginalized in our society and the immigration system from participating in literary and research efforts focused on their situation.

Equally relevant, children might lack the skills to tell their stories as well as a critical understanding of their own situation. Not only they are often small children, but they have also escaped violence and poverty, experienced a dangerous and long trip, are confused on being detained, do not know how long they will be detained, and feel lonely and miss their loved ones. For example, Luis was only seven or 8-year old, and Jeremias was sixteen when they were detained. Although they had distinct coping mechanisms, neither had sufficient English skills to speak for themselves. Denying them of the use of the first language in the centers only aggravated their trauma and their fear. Despite the hard conditions they experienced, Luis and Jeremias were expected to learn English and communicate in this language, which only created harder paths and destinies for them, and made them ultimately unable to tell their stories as they would have in their mother tongue.[3]

Critically, changing details also protects the service providers, who may depend on their employment within or in collaboration with immigration and detention systems for their livelihood. Working and volunteering in these environments can be particularly challenging when the political climate is highly charged on the topic of immigration. Further, service providers are often bound by their employer's policies, professional ethical codes, and personal moral standings to avoid identifying any of the clients they serve. Indeed, *Serving Refugee Children* specifically changes some data in order to comply with confidentiality agreements providers sign in order to be able to serve refugee children and avoid any violations of their privacy.

Contributing authors have sometimes spent years working with immigrant children and have listened to their traumatic experiences. Working and volunteering in the centers deeply affected contributors, who rethought approaches for listening, healing, and offering solidarity to children. The Director of the Centre for the Study of Storytelling, Experientiality, and Memory at the University of Turku, Finland, Hanna Meretoja asserts, "the condition of genuine solidarity is the ability to refrain from taking the other as the same as oneself: it is to acknowledge commonality, while at the same time being sensitive to the differences between the I and the non-I."[4] Diana Tietjens Meyers cites Serene Khader's advice on how to interview victims so that, in doing so, interviewers discern the particularity of the victim, apprehend their needs that might be in conflict with their own, and immerse themselves in the victim's circumstances.[5] For providers, serving refugee chilren involved humility to listening to the painful facts that disconcerted them. Their accounts detail how much providers and volunteers cared and the limitations in caring and serving imposed by the realities of their jobs and roles. Their struggles make obvious that policies in place are not designed for refugee children.

However, listening was often the first step to solace, solidarity, and action for them.[6] Being listened to may be even more crucial for the emotional wellbeing of isolated and lonely refugees and detainees. In those moments of expressing courage, hope, determination, resiliency, and spirit, life was experienced as meaningful. Meretoja explains, "we are constituted by storytelling, by sharing our lives and experiences with others, and that this is so indispensable for human existence that the inability to engage in storytelling—closing up into silence and muteness—can lead to something worse than death: the complete erosion of the self."[7] Listening is indeed a powerful force in shaping our sense of self and in human relationships. Texts show this obvious affective dimension of the act of sharing their life experiences while in these centers and schools. We hope that the act of telling their stories created a relational space that soothed children while in detention.

By sharing with the general public their working and volunteering experiences with Camila, Carlos, Danny Mateo, Jeremías, Luz, Luis, Juan, Sheila, Toñito, William, and Ximena, contributors show how they tried to find ways to listen and express solidarity. As Diana Tietjens Meyers states,

> victims of human rights abuse are routinely silenced. Their stories are told, if they are told at all, only in private settings. Consequently, they do not come to the attention of the public. Suppressing victims' stories is a form of revictimization. It compounds the harms that the victims have already endured by condemning them to isolation from the larger moral community.[8]

In doing so, authors contribute to building a culture of human rights that listens to victims' perspectives and lessens their suffering.

The importance of ethically uncovering these individual stories for policy change cannot be overstated. Our contributors are in the unique position of collecting a plurality of experiences from children who are largely marginalized and rejected in contemporary American society and politics. According to Patricia Ewick and Susan Silbey, "subversive stories do not aggregate to the general, do not collect particulars as examples of a common phenomenon or rule; rather subversive stories recount particular experiences as rooted and part of an encompassing cultural, material, and political word."[9] For instance, official reports may say that Jeremías was a violent child and had to be sent to a high-security prison. They might even report that Luis was successfully placed with a close relative. Retamales's and Lupe's narrations on Jeremías and Luis say otherwise. They detail the emotions shared while the children were under their care and the regulations that caused great pain to both children. In other words, service providers make visible the explicit connections between the particular experience of children and the inhumane conditions dictated by policies. Similarly, Luz was assumed to be a member of MS-13. However, Michelson, who spent hours with her in poetry workshops documents that she was instead a victim of the gang. Effective listening therefore builds on intentional care. The same child's story is interpreted totally differently when listened to by a caring provider in the comforting surroundings of writing poems or painting pictures, than by a special investigator—with not enough Spanish and humanistic skills—in a room with no windows and fluorescent lights.

The solidarity and care expressed by authors are practices of resistance that struggle against forces seeking to silence and isolate migrant children. Listening and dialoguing with the victims of violence are necessary steps towards the exercise of solidarity, and ultimately social justice.[10] In those acts of conversation between children and service providers, and in the resulting texts and translations in *Serving Refugee Children*, we wish to collectively bridge children's isolation and stand in solidarity with them. To heal the historical wounds that underlie our current immigration crisis, society needs to listen to its victims.

Distressingly, our hope is symbolic of our service. For the most part, service providers who care for children in a detention center, a school for newcomers, or a medical setting do not get to know the whereabouts and outcomes of refugee children. Stories featured in this collection reflect this reality. Serving them means contending with the fear that deportation, criminalization, and trauma are very likely to be present in their lives. Serving Refugee Children aims to foster the recollection of stories by courageous and hopeful children, otherwise silenced.

Storytelling engages writers and readers at an emotional level, allowing them "to interpret the realm of the possible with imaginative reasoning."[11] Meretoja states,

> If ethical understanding is a phoretic art that cannot be taught in abstraction and that is characterized by the temporal process of experiencing and imagining concrete situations in their complexity, it is no wonder that narrative fiction -which is emphatically about temporal process of ethical decision-making in complex fictional worlds- is the art of ethical imagination ... The most important contribution of narrative fiction to ethical imagination takes place when the application of knowledge that we already possess is precisely not enough.[12]

Other fields of knowledge speak in the past or present tense seeking to generalize experiences and truths for policy making. To the contrary, storytelling, "allow[s] us to think in the subjunctive mode, as sociologist Robin Wagner-Pacifici puts it."[13] That is to say, it goes beyond responding "who, what, when, and why." By appealing to readers' emotions storytelling asks "what if" and helps listeners and readers imagine otherwise, it makes sense of experience, channels emotions, sustains collective action, and "it allows us to glimpse alternative possibilities and their likely consequences."[14]

According to Meretoja, storytelling

"can nourish an ethos of dialogue that makes us more responsive to one another's wounds and vulnerabilities, as well as to the ways in which we are implicated in violent histories that we have inherited, histories in which we silently or actively participate, or against which we struggle. Narratives driven by such an ethos have the potential to create a transsubjective narrative in-between that opens up pathways to less violent futures."[15]

Similarly, Meyers remind us that stories of victims and stories of those who help victims are a matter of human rights and common humanity, "although the human rights regime is founded on the value of our common humanity, in practice implicit biases divide us into valued and disvalued social groups and subvert our commitment to the value of common humanity."[16] Stories here represent common humanity and subvert favorable official reports on abusive policies and dehumanizing narratives of immigrants.

In response to the postmodernist critique of narrative as a coherent system of representation, Meretoja asserts, "it is simplistic and reductionist to reject all attempts at understanding as inherently violent."[17] Stories show bonds between providers and children amidst lack of institutional support for the wellbeing of refugees. In the stories presented here, readers get to know the emotions of children as well as service providers. Often, they shared many emotions and became friends, other times they had to be strong for the children and provide them hope. With their dedication, contributors became important people in the lives of refugee children. However, they were often unable to avoid the pain caused by the policies in place.

Contributors and editors advocate for first-person narratives and for changes in legislation that would allow unaccompanied youth to tell their detention stories in their first language and with trained personnel. In the interim, *Serving Refugee Children* bears witness. Contributing authors' portrayals are reliable and intentionally humanistic and did not write "fiction masquerading as fact."[18] Following Meretoja, editors believe that storytelling is one of the ethical ways to engage with the experiences of the very vulnerable protagonists in this collection. Meyers claims that in order to respect "the integrity and complexity of victims' stories" requires that victims "should not be reduced to passive, helpless, dehumanized cyphers when their stories are used to promote human rights."[19] In *Serving Refugee Children*, readers equally learn about the youth's courage, solidarity, faith, and capacity to trust, and not only about the discriminatory circumstances they encounter.

Storytelling is employed here as an effective method of producing and acquiring knowledge and empathy. It cultivates readers' awareness and openness to multiple perspectives, a necessary condition for ethical inquiry and agency. Polletta argues that precisely because stories are open to multiple interpretations, "they better capture particularity than universality and concreteness rather than abstraction."[20] Diversity is precisely what storytelling claims, rather than universal or absolute truths. Ewick and Silbey explain, "the political commitment to giving voice and bearing witness through narrative is underwritten by the epistemological conviction that there is no single, objective apprehensive truth."[21] Beyond encompassing a culture of human rights in which each victim's story is important, storytelling makes evident the narrowness and errors in the supposedly general understandings that constitute policies. As Ewick and Silbey claim, "narratives have the capacity to reveal truths about the social world that are flattened or silenced by an insistence on more traditional methods of social science and legal scholarship."[22] By its particular, emotional, imaginative reasoning, and diversity, contributors "bring human rights down from the empyrean of mathematical and moral abstraction, and by sparking empathetic engagement with individual targeted for human abuse, promote awareness of the paramount urgency of securing human rights."[23]

Contributing authors are aware of their own interpretative mediation as well as the children's selective memory. Editors have applied Meretoja's hermeneutic narrative ethics as a framework to analytically evaluate their narrative practices. They have reflected about their own biases in order to make sure they do not misinform the public or minimize or maximize events. As authors, they understand their responsibility but also ask readers to consider narrative hermeneutics, which "treats narratives as culturally mediated practices" of (re)interpreting experience and articulates how storytelling can function as a non-totalizing mode of responding to the stories' singularity.[24] In this regard, Meretoja proposes seeing "interpretation as an endless activity of (re)orientation, engagement, and sense-making."[25] Contributors share their own emotions in trying to navigate policies that are designed for menacing individuals instead of vulnerable children. Despite these difficult regulations, they were able to show their care, dedication, and admiration for these strong and adaptable refugee children.

By narrating stories of resistance, *Serving Refugee Children* aims to foster a culture of empathy that may ultimately change present inhumane conditions for refuge-seeking children. Meyers believes that empathy can transform value systems and policies, "what attuned empathetic engagement with a victim's story can accomplish is to bring a reader or auditor close enough to a victim for the addressee to grasp the colossal disvalue of human rights abuse, irrespective of who is undergoing it."[26] The news, reports, and statistics might desensitize the public about the plight of refugees and reinforce negative stereotypes about them. Instead, their stories, told by workers and activists working with them, engage readers to imagine what is like to live with the biased perceptions of refugees and the discrimination and suffering they endure. Editors and authors evidence the need for institutional reform the need for institutional reform. These subversive stories are told with the aim of undermining official reports and their silencing of children's pain.

On Previous Publications

Children's books have long chronicled refugee families' journeys, separations, and deportations (Anzaldúa 1993; Colato Laínez 2004, 2010; Alvarez 2010; Resau 2012; Kim 2013; Mateo 2014; Buitrago 2015; Danticat 2015). Most recently, Jorge Argueta's *We Are Like the Clouds/Somos Como las Nubes* (2016), a bilingual collection of poems, is addressed to children ages 7 to 12. Refugee minors often speak of what they left behind and their fears for the future. Several bilingual publications have portrayed the migration journeys of children, either alone or accompanied; for instance, Alfredo Alva's *La frontera: El viaje con papá* (2018), Yuyi Morales' *Soñadores* (2018); Jairo Buitrago's *Dos conejos blancos* (2016); Alexandra Díaz's *El único destino* (2016); and Amanda Irma Pérez's *My Diary from Here to There* (2002).

Similarly, stories of migrant children with their undocumented families and friends have also been widely anthologized; some have become classics of the U.S. Latino literary canon, among them stand out Tomás Rivera's *. . . y no se lo tragó la tierra* (1971), Sandra Cisneros's *The House on Mango Street* (1984), and Francisco Jiménez's *The Circuit: Stories from the Life of a Migrant Child* (1997) and *Breaking Through* (2001), and Javier Zamora *Unaccompanied* (2017). Importantly, these texts, while only 15- to 20-year old, predate major shifts in immigration trends that occurred in 2015 and 2016. As subsequent sections of this introduction will elucidate, Central American migration to the U.S. became largely a matter of family and child migration—often times characterized by the migration of children without any adult guardian—in 2015–2016. Previous publications cannot speak to the experiences of service providers, or the reality of childhood detention, following the surge in family and child migration that occurred in 2015–2016 and continues today.

These critically acclaimed books disseminate children's heart-wrenching accounts of migration and undocumented life in the U.S. However, fewer works have focused on the perspective of service providers and allies of unaccompanied children as detainees—likely due to the aforementioned barriers in seeking permission for publishing case reports—and none, to our knowledge, have sought the perspective of the people who care for these children in the U.S. Published in 2015, Susan Terrio's *Whose Child Am I? Unaccompanied, Undocumented Children in U.S. Immigration Custody* masterfully blends personal narratives from interviews with undocumented youth with archival research on immigration law and reports on the U.S. Custom and Border Protection programs where undocumented minors are detained. In 2017, Seth Michelson's *Dreaming America* recovers the stories of detained youth for all audiences. Michelson, one of the contributors to *Serving Refugee Children* conducted poetry workshops in two detention centers for undocumented, unaccompanied youth (13–17 years of age) in the U.S. His bilingual collection features 41 Spanish poems and their English translations. *Serving Refugee Children* continues this legacy by advocating for the abolition of current detention practices, with the hope that this multi-genre envisions humane and safe prison practices.

Professor of Law César Cuauhtémoc García Hernández claims that lawyers and organizers have tried to reform immigration detention in the past but ultimately institutions have solidified their practice and created harsher conditions. In the concluding chapter of his book, *Migrating to Prison*, García Hernández reviews several initiatives that have worked in the past and would make prison reform successful. He claims that they are mostly not in practice because of the deeply ingrained negative stereotypes about Hispanic immigrants as a national thread or as wandering foreign souls with no deep ties to the U.S. The editors and contributors of this collection believe that sharing accounts about immigrants can help solve this root cause—prejudice and indifference about the suffering of others.[27]

On Terminology

The works in *Serving Refugee Children*, in their terminology, reflect the variety of words and phrases (and implied opinions) used for immigrant minors in the U.S. At the most general level, once a foreign-born person settles in the U.S., they have "an immigrant" status. They can become a citizen, a lawful permanent resident, a refugee, an asylum seeker, or an undocumented immigrant.[28] The U.S. Citizenship and Immigration Services (i.e., USCIS) defines a documented immigrant as someone who has been granted the right to reside permanently in the U.S., also known as a lawful permanent resident. An undocumented immigrant, on the other hand, is someone who entered the U.S. without the proper legal authorization or entered the U.S. with legal authorization but violated the terms of the visa status. According to The United Nations High Commission on Refugees (UNHCR), a main difference between immigrants and refugees is that immigrants choose to move to the U.S., not because of a direct threat of persecution or death, as in the case of refugees, but mainly to improve their lives (e.g., financially, educationally, due to family reunion, or other reasons).[29] Thus, a refugee is defined as a person fleeing natural disaster, armed conflict, or persecution based on race, religion, nationality, or political opinion.[30]

In a technical sense, Central American youth are usually not refugees, as they do not seek or receive refugee status prior to migration. Instead, Central American youth and families often pursue an asylum process after arriving at the U.S. border. An asylum seeker is someone who claims to be a refugee but has not yet had his or her case evaluated or accepted. Seeking asylum is, and has been, a right protected in Article 14 of the United Nations' Universal Declaration of Human Rights for 70 years (UN, 1948). To qualify for asylum in the U.S., applicants must demonstrate that (1) they fear persecution, (2) the persecution would occur based on race, religion, nationality, political opinion, or social group, and (3) that the home country government is either involved in the persecution or unable to control it.[31]

Finally, the U.S. Homeland Security Act of 2002 (Homeland Security, 2002) defines unaccompanied minors as children who have no lawful immigration status in the U.S., have not attained 18 years of age, and have no parent or legal guardian available to provide care and physical custody in the U.S. Upon apprehension, unaccompanied immigrant children are temporarily detained by border patrol officers from the Department of Homeland Security (i.e., DHS). Many children are then placed in the Unaccompanied Refugee Minors Program operated by the Office of Refugee Resettlement (ORR). Minors are placed in a shelter facility, foster care or group home, or other special needs facilities based on a number of considerations including trafficking, mental health needs, criminal background, and age.[32] The ORR facilities have a legal responsibility to ensure that unaccompanied minors receive a full range of assistance including shelter, counseling, medical care, and legal services. For instance, medical services (which include mental health screening) must be provided within 48 hours of admission.[33] If evaluation and/or observation suggest that another placement would better meet the child's needs, care providers must make transfer recommendations within 3 days after identifying the need for a transfer.[34] Critically, while children are held in ORR, there is ambiguity surrounding who their legal guardian is.

Despite the aforementioned ORR policies meant to protect children while in custody and move children rapidly out of detention and into facilities that meet their needs, concerns regarding improper treatment of children in the immigration system as a whole have been reported. For example, according to the Women's Refugee Commission, the conditions at CBP facilities (though not ORR facilities) are often inhumane, degrading, and frightening for children. For instance, the holding cells are extremely cold, windowless, and lined with fluorescent lights which are on 24 hours a day.[35] Moreover, children lack access to showers and appropriate spaces for recreation. Many of the minors have also complained that they are not provided with enough food to eat or water to drink. Finally, the facilities are so crowded that children have to take turns laying on the concrete floor to sleep. Detention centers might be run by for-profit corporations that often fall short on standards for safety and wellbeing.[36] Advocacy organizations have reported that children are detained in CBP facilities longer than 72 hours.[37]

Another challenge experienced by unaccompanied minors in the U.S. is the lack of legal representation because children lack the financial resources or the connections with pro-bono attorneys to attain representation.[38] Indeed, current policy allows unaccompanied children to represent themselves in immigration court with no legal aid.[39] Moreover, the stressors associated with detention, such as fear, anxiety, and frustration, can exacerbate preexisting mental health conditions.[40] The *Washington Post* published that the number of migrant children held without their parents by the U.S. government surged 21% in 2018 as a result of the new policy, and there was a total of 10,773 children detained in May 2018, which included children who had crossed the border unaccompanied.[41]. All of these recent developments have increased the number of immigrant children in the United Sates without legal guardianship—thereby increasing the population of children with experiences to be represented but with no parental/legal permission to participate in sharing their traumatic experiences.

The Trump Administration sought to lessen concerns about these children but released little or no information to the public or the federal government on their whereabouts. Visits to the detention centers were also monitored.[42]

Recent research shows limited legal counsel has important implications for immigrant minors. For instance, during the 2017 fiscal year, 94% of immigrant minors without legal counsel who had their case decided in immigration court were forced to return to their home country, while 45% of immigrant minors with legal counsel were allowed to remain in the U.S.[43]

In 2017, 41,435 *new* "unaccompanied alien children" were apprehended by U.S. border patrol at the U.S./Mexico Border.[44] In 2016, 59,692 unaccompanied adolescents were taken into custody at the U.S./Mexico border.[45] The Office of Refugee Resettlement places many in the care of family, friends, or a foster parent while they await immigration court hearings determining their eligibility for special protections, asylum, and other relief from deportation. While many may qualify for relief from deportation, immigrant adolescents are not provided free legal counsel, may not speak English, and are unfamiliar with the U.S. legal system, providing them little hope (Pair Project, n.d.); indeed, less than 10% are actually granted relief from removal.[46]

The large increases in youth migration to the U.S. from Central America—particularly El Salvador, Guatemala, and Honduras—are largely driven by crime, death, and violence in those countries, having reached record levels in the last 5 years. Indeed, the increases in regional violence predate the large increase in unaccompanied minors migrating to the U.S. that occurred in 2014 and 2015, with Honduras reporting the highest homicide rate globally in 2011; 2013 marking the end of a truce between major gang powers in El Salvador; and crime victimization cited as a major reason for Central American migration in 2014.[47] Violence in the region has continued and, in turn, continues to motivate migration to the U.S. As the socio-political climate of Central America has changed, so have patterns of Hispanic immigration to the U.S. Between 2015 and 2016 alone, there was a 131% increase in the number of children and families crossing the Southwestern border of the U.S., reflecting large numbers of families seeking "humanitarian protection."[48]

Despite changes in immigration policy designed to stem this flow, family apprehensions at the Southwestern U.S. border fell only 2.6% percent between 2016 and 2017, indicating that high rates of family migration have become the norm, rather than the exception. In turn, dramatic increases in rates of crime, violence, and death in Central America have corresponded to increases in reports of trauma and post-traumatic symptoms among recent waves of Hispanic immigrants.[49] The immigrant experiences captured in *Serving Refugee Children* document this reality—the prototypic experience of risking life and death alone during migration in order to flee danger and ultimately reach a nation in which your right to enter, remain, or receive protection from the adversities of your home country are contested by policy and popular opinion.

Historical Context

The forces that have pushed migrants out of Central America in recent years are steeped in a historical context that involves the U.S. from the outset and, in fact, reaches back several decades. The population of Central American immigrants in the U.S. rose most sharply in the 1980s when it more than tripled, due to political and economic forces in Central America,[50] though since the 1950s, these same forces had been at play in Central American migration.[51] It is important to note that the civil wars that motivated migratory flows in the 1980s and 1990s involved the U.S. directly. Alvarado, Estrada, & Hernández provide a summary of U.S. intervention in the Northern Triangle region of Central America (i.e., Honduras, El Salvador, and Guatemala) in their edited volume.[52] They cite U.S. involvement in El Salvador's civil war, including assistance with air bombings and continued U.S. military funding in the midst of a deeply violent civil war. They further juxtapose this military involvement with the U.S. immigration response during and immediately after the war—denying asylum to Salvadoran migrants to the U.S. who fled such violence, defining them as economic migrants rather than refugees.

Likewise, Guatemalan history includes U.S. sponsored dictatorships and interventions dating back decades including a military coup d'état by the U.S. which was ultimately followed by dictatorships which "created the conditions that fueled the thirty-six-year civil war" in Guatemala. The effects of the 36-year civil war that followed were devastating; more than 45,000 individuals who disappeared and 200,000 killed, with most of this destruction occurring through state sponsored violence, and much of which was genocidal towards individuals of Mayan ethnicity. Though former President Bill Clinton officially apologized for the U.S.'s role in the civil war in 1999, U.S. immigration policies remained out of sync, largely denying Guatemalans legal entry or refugee status. Guatemalans and Salvadorans in the U.S. continue to make up a large portion of undocumented migrants in the U.S., in contrast to Nicaraguans and Cubans who were favored in immigration policy following war and instability in those countries.

Throughout the aforementioned conflicts and others in the region, including Nicaragua, the U.S. utilized Honduras as an ally, ultimately engaging in military intervention in Honduras as well. It is notable that the

U.S.-CIA-trained Battalion 3–16 in Honduras "is closely linked to both the proliferation of *maras* [gangs] in twenty-first century Honduras and in influencing the national police, who rule corruptly and with total impunity, contributing to Honduras being named today as one of the most dangerous and deadliest nations in the Western Hemisphere."[53] Like other Northern Triangle migrants, Honduran immigrants to the U.S. were largely seen as economic migrants and did not benefit from systematic asylum or refuge immigration policies following regional violence. In contrast, instability in the region caused by Hurricane Mitch, which struck Central America in 1998, and killed approximately 18,000 people. Honduras experienced the greatest devastation, resulting in a Temporary Protected Status program in immigration policy that registered 64,000 Hondurans after the hurricane. No such policies have acknowledged the reality that U.S. intervention in Central America is responsible, in part, for the instability that prompted—and continues to prompt—migrant flows. Alvarado, Estrada, and Hernández (2017) summarize their discussion of U.S. intervention in Central America writing that "recent migration trends are intrinsically connected to the economic, political, and military strategies the United States planned and then deployed onto Central America . . . [which] shaped Central American poverty and the disenfranchisement of marginalized peoples."

Robert Lovato, a journalist specializing in Central America and recipient of a Pulitzer grant, connects the aforementioned involvement of the U.S. in Central America to current crises of violence, gang activity, and migration in the region. Indeed, battalion forces that were initially trained by the U.S. CIA are now the same forces being used by the government in attempts to control gang activity;[54] El Salvador is currently the battleground for two major gang powers, 18th Street Gang and Mara Salvatrucha (MS). Further, Lovato quotes Salvadorans who assert that the U.S. was part of the military and political activities that destroyed the social fabric of El Salvador, leaving a vacancy that was then occupied by gangs.[55] The same assertion has been made regarding the results of U.S. intervention in other Central American nations as well. In practical terms, the arms and military training left over after conflicts in the region made guns widely available after the civil wars had officially ended.[56] Availability of military skill and weaponry facilitated the rapid growth of armed gangs.

Moreover, critical analyses of the current situation in Central America continue to site the U.S. as a contributor to violence in the region, beyond historic intervention efforts. For instance, the highlights that Central America and the U.S. are inextricably, geographically linked via the drug trade, with the U.S. being the largest consumer of illicit drugs and Central America being the thoroughfare between that consumer and the producers in South America.[57] While U.S. policies have historically targeted suppliers of illicit drugs in South America, they do less to invest in reducing the demand for illicit drugs in the U.S., and thus, supply markets continue to exist and funnel drugs through Central America. Likewise, ample scholarship suggests that the most prominent Central American gangs, MS and 18th Street, were actually formed in U.S. cities and only exported to Central America in the last 20 years as a result of deportations linked to the Illegal Immigration Reform and Immigrant Responsibility Act of 1996.[58] In concert with the disenfranchisement of Central Americans caused by decades of war and political instability, the arrival of gang-active-deportees to Central America allowed for the rapid growth of gangs in the region.[59] Immigration policies in the U.S. continue to prioritize deportation of immigrants who have acquired criminal records in the U.S., continuing the flow of individuals with criminal sentiments and limited options for meaningful alternatives to crime in the Northern Triangle region.

Serving Refugee Children represents, to varying extents, this historical context. They address, head on, gang violence and government corruption in Central America and, though the historical context of these forces may not feature in the narratives of children, it cannot be forgotten. Without this context, it may appear that Central Americans are inherently fraught with criminality or chaos—falsehoods that evaporate when considering the varied historical and current forces that continue to subjugate the nations of the Northern Triangle. Likewise, accounts, in some cases, show the hopes of migrants seeking the elusive American Dream. These aspirations, while common in refugee children, stand in contrast with the experiences of many Central Americans who rightly view the U.S. as the source of much injustice in their region (e.g., the birthplace of prominent gangs) and the experiences of many individuals deported from their attempt at the American Dream. This historical and current context cannot be forgotten when reading the stories collected in *Serving Refugee Children*.

Organization and Format

Serving Refugee Children show the perils children face on their journeys to safety and in immigration detention through a combination of genres—short narratives, reflections, poetry, memoirs, and testimonials. For some of the contributors, storytelling came as a helpful way to express their relationship with unaccompanied minors; for others, it was poetry that best captured their experiences. Finally, other contributors chose essays. As editors, we welcomed any genre that served the aim of denouncing the children's ordeals.

Specifically, *Serving Refugee Children* features services providers' interactions with children from Honduras, El Salvador, Mexico, and other Central American countries, with ages between 7- and 18-years old. Linguistically speaking, the richness of several Spanish varieties and code-switching in an English-only context articulate the grassroots and transnational nature of supporting refugee children. Although editors have striven for a general standard variety of Spanish, they have been mindful to maintain the Spanish variety of the child. Original texts are followed by translations that care for bilingual and bicultural readers interested in Latinx youth migration to the U.S. In this respect, bilingualism in *Serving Refugee Children* is a non-totalizing mode of listening and understanding diverse perspectives and help readers acknowledge commonality while being open to differences.

As editors, we have not necessarily strived for uniform literary quality. We were disturbed by the candor of some accounts and wanted to preserve their truth. The sometimes-rough quality of some pieces is telling of the alarming situations these children are in and speak to the fact they are helped by volunteers and service providers with diverse backgrounds and approaches. *Serving Refugee Children* renders coming of age stories within the context of extreme survival decisions, dehumanizing processes, and desperate conditions. One of the strengths of this anthology lies in its diversity of genres, perspectives, and professional experiences that allows for accessible format and writing style for the general reader.

Serving Refugee Children offers powerful themes, such as violence, access to justice, assimilation, criminalization of immigration, dehumanization, processes of othering, the impact of detention on families and communities, nostalgia, psychological harm, solution-driven narratives, uncertainty, and the fight for good standards for wellbeing and treatment, as well as resilience and healing. Four sections organize these themes and narrate the tragic migrations of children who leave their homes in Central America, often alone, and to seek refuge in the U.S.

Part I, "Escapes and Crossings," portrays narratives about the unaccompanied minors' reasons for escaping from danger and risking their lives on the journey. These reasons include high rates of crime, gang and cartel related violence, and poverty. Ultimately, unaccompanied minors reach the U.S. after a dangerous, long migration journey that includes the most abject and desperate conditions (treacherous landscapes, extreme temperatures, little or no food and water), all of which make them extremely vulnerable.

This first section opens with, "Looking for Luz," by Seth Michelson, who met Luz during his poetry workshop in a restrictive detention center on the East Coast. Michelson met numerous incarcerated children while leading his writing workshops. He vividly remembers Luz's indomitable spirit as she told him her story of emergency escape from violence in El Salvador to incarceration in the U.S. Luz is now in an isolation cell in a maximum-security detention center as an undocumented, unaccompanied minor. The story celebrates her courage and determination. Wendy Herrera translates the story into Spanish.

"Looking for Luz" is followed by Paloma Villegas' poem "Los niños floreros," and its translation into English. It depicts Villegas's own crossing of the border with her brother as minors without state required documents two decades ago. This narrative focuses on the processes through which borders felt almost as crusts in the children's bodies.

The first part ends with Cassandra Bailey's "Growing Up Too Fast," which narrates a common account confided to the author while she was providing psychological services to unaccompanied immigrant youth in shelters in Texas from 2016 to 2018. Similar to other young girls who are victims of gang violence, the story about Ximena's coming of age as an undocumented immigrant in the U.S. stands in contrast to the images she saw on television while in El Salvador of carefree *gringas*. The narrative reveals tension between the desires of a common adolescent girl and the demands placed on a recent immigrant who needs to prioritize survival. Betsy E. Garcia translates the story into Spanish.

In Part II, "Memories and Bonds," three texts examine the complexities surrounding the unprocessed emotions and haunting memories these very vulnerable minors experience once in the U.S. These stories portray early separation from family members, uprooting from familiar contexts of language and culture, poor physical or mental health, and exposure to violence.

Melissa Briones, Alfonso Mercado, Abigail Nunez-Saenz, Paola Quijano, and Andy Torres write the first piece of creative narrative, "Buscando un destino" (Searching for a Destiny/Destination), which shows the bonding between a boy from El Salvador, Toñito, and his young mother, Marta. The authors composed this hopeful account as a way to express their frustration with the dehumanizing process that many immigrants suffer. As volunteers at the Humanitarian Respite Center in South Texas, Melissa Briones, Paola Quijao, Andy Torres, Abigail Nunez-Saenz and Dr. Alfonso Mercado assisted undocumented immigrant families released by government officials and dropped off at a bus station. In search of their sponsors, migrants often find themselves lost in an unknown country and immersed in a language they do not speak. Volunteers offer guidance to immigrants and refugees, a warm meal, clean clothes, toiletries, medicines they may need, and a place to spend the night if needed. The narrative centers on the theme of solidarity found in respite centers. As Wendy Vogt states migrant shelters are spaces "of refuge in a larger matrix of migration and survival." They are "node[s] in a national and transnational network of solidarity and resistance."[60] The story switches from Spanish to English, language usage that is common in the U.S./Mexico border region. An English translation is added.

The second piece in this section, Yessica Colin's "Camila" tells the story of an undocumented 16-year old adolescent attending an American school. The author recently worked for 2 years as a research assistant in a school in Texas that admitted and helped immigrants. Yessica conducted one-on-one interviews and was deeply affected by the story of Camila, a young Nicaraguan woman who had recently left her native land. Camila confided to the Yessica her determination to provide for her brother. The story contrasts Camila's psychological burden of leaving her brother behind with her commitment to provide him with a safe future. The piece's unique perspective relates to the many reasons why undocumented minors and adolescents flee their home countries in search of a better life, despite the odds and the sadness at leaving behind family. Wendy Herrera translates the story into Spanish.

The last piece, Ana Maria Fores Tamayo's poem, "Elegy to a Refugee Girl," and its translation into Spanish portrays a recent interaction between a teacher and a 7-year-old child talking about her painting in the Pro Se asylum clinic where Fores Tamayo provides services in Texas. For the author, her poem is an allegory for marginalized women and children. This narrative, then, pays tribute to the women and children she has helped through the asylum pro se clinic.[61]

Part III, "Silencing," further depicts barriers and additional challenges in adjusting to the U.S. Children may face racial discrimination and the uncertainty of their immigration status and consequent detention. The first piece by Maria Baños Jordan, "Spanish Silencio" considers linguistic and cultural barriers in human interaction. This poem was created during a workshop with 25 girls in the Conroe Historias Biography Book Project in Texas.

The poem speaks of what is lost in translation when newcomers learn English, but their culture is not equally acknowledged. In "Spanish Silencio," the author captures young women's frustration as they hope to be heard beyond their imperfect usage of English language and be seen as worthy individuals with much to give. Wendy Herrera translates the poem into Spanish.

Francisco Villegas and Paloma Villegas's "Reflection on schooling experiences as undocumented migrants in the U.S" describe their own schooling experience in the 1990s. They remark how, as undocumented children, school felt like a psychological border because they suffered fears of deportation, lack of proper access to resources, and bullying.

Estrella Godinez's "A Yearning Desire" follows the path of a young boy, Danny Mateo, who finds it hard to adapt to the U.S. until a Christian group helps him. Godinez met him while interviewing recently immigrated Central Americans in a school for immigrant youth in Texas from 2016 to 2018. A supporter of refugee's rights, Estrella was inspired by young Danny Mateo's determination to fight for a better life.

"Jeremías" by Jaime Retamales completes this section sharing the experience of Jeremías, a child who escaped Honduras looking for a safer environment. Retamales, a legal assistant volunteer and teacher in an immigrant shelter and high security center in Texas, taught Jeremías for 6 months in 2015. Ultimately, this piece of creative nonfiction is about broken dreams and how detention centers fail many undocumented children. Tara Marshall translates the story into English.

Part IV, "The Love of Strangers" continues with the theme of protecting minors by recognizing the ethics of professionals working in detention centers and schools. These inspiring professionals think about creative ways to support refugee children. They often find themselves in the position of having to choose between compliance with state law and professional or individual ethics. This conflict places individual agencies and social workers in extremely difficult positions, and often at odds. These stories testify to how often immigrant children are in most need of empathy, compassion, and supportive mental health services rather than detention and imprisonment.

The section opens with Luz M. Garcini and Martin La Roche's "An Undocumented Journey in Search of a Heart." The authors, who are medical providers, write the account of their relationship with Juan, an undocumented 18-year old adolescent at a hospice in California, where the authors provided him with palliative care in 2014. Told from a perspective of a medical provider, this story provides insight into Juan's strengths, struggles, and coping mechanisms, in hopes of inciting reflection that can help society move beyond walls and borders. Many of these walls are not only being built in the southern border but are cultural and contextual constructs that divide people according to skin color, socioeconomic status or place of birth. At a time in which many are being forgotten or stigmatized, it is important to know their stories. Mercedes Fernández Asenjo translates the story into Spanish.

The next piece, "An ESL Classroom as a Healing Space," by Juan A. Ríos Vega draws on critical race theory (CRT) and Latino Critical Theory (LatCrit) to reflect on his journey teaching undocumented immigrant students (16–18 years of age) in a middle and high school in the Southeast from 1999 to 2012. Although the ESL classroom can be a site of struggle for learners, Ríos Vega's experience demonstrates the importance of providing safe spaces that allow students to develop trust and resilience. Montse Feu translates the reflection into Spanish.

The last piece, "The Love of Strangers," by Amelia Cotter portrays the relationship between a young Mexican boy, Luis, and Lupe, an immigrant detention worker in Texas in 2016. Because Lupe at the detention center did not want to be identified, the story is written by author Amelia Cotter. The story covers a different aspect of the relationship between workers and detained children, that of minors who are searching for pillars of love and affection and become attached to adults and authority figures around them during their journeys through the legal system. Blanca P. Tovar Frias translates the story into Spanish.

Current legislation and bureaucracy limit first-person narratives. Service providers authoring the pieces in *Serving Refugee Children* are personally affected and directly impacted by this current legislation in the midst of the immigration crisis in the border. Through the power of telling stories, *Serving Refugee Children* exposes current detention center and school conditions while also protecting refugee children. Morally obliged to share their experiences, authors have embraced storytelling, poetry, and essay writing as a means for social change. In this regard, they advocate for accountability in detention facilities and paths for citizenship for refugee minors.

One of the outcomes of *Serving Refugee Children* is the practice of rehumanization. Luz and Jeremías's stories, for instance, show how current anti-immigrant rhetoric dehumanizes migrants. Because of this type of rhetoric, children who seek refuge are often identified as MS-13 members or as threats to the U.S. in an anti-immigrant paradigm.[62] In contrast, Seth Michelson and Jaime Retamales listen to the children's stories and nurture their relationships with them. Their unflinching accounts of children's realities shine a light on the forces that compel children to flee their homes and families while risking their own lives in search of safety and prosperity in the U.S.

Also, *Serving Refugee Children* shows the struggles and traumatic experiences that children undergo when seeking safety in the U.S., and find instead imprisonment, separation from their families, and ICE raids in what would have become their neighborhoods. "The Elegy of a Refugee Girl" and "Spanish Silencio" are the stories of courageous children that proclaim the strength of survivors. Most importantly, these stories reenact the potential of asylum seekers, refugees, and migrants. Toñito and Marta, Camila and Charly, and Paloma and Francisco Villegas defeat the perception that migrants are passive victims of their lives, and, instead show their resilient leadership in becoming powerful agents of change in their communities.

Serving Refugee Children sheds light to the powerful role of religion as a coping mechanism for some protagonists. Juan's and Danny Mateo's heart-wrenching accounts of death and survival powerfully describe what it is like to resist, learn, love, provide, pray, and blossom in two languages, amidst dire circumstances and dehumanizing processes. Likewise, stories told in the mother tongue prove to be indispensable to human survival. Toñito and Ximena illustrate how many migrants see the world in two or more languages, and Luis and Jeremias draw as a way of expression since their Spanish language has been forbidden for them to use. The poem "Spanish Silencio" poeticizes silence as the erosion of the self when we are forced to communicate in other than the native language. Sheila, William, and Carlos, like most of the protagonists in this anthology experience storytelling as a healing and resistance practice in detention facilities, respite centers, hospices, and schools.

In fact, *Serving Refugee Children* seeks to illustrate two dominant theoretical approaches in immigration research within the social sciences: the tension between resilience and risk present in the immigrant paradox and the broader task of acculturation universal in the immigrant experience. The immigrant paradox, a framework often utilized to conceptualize findings from medical and social science studies of immigrants, suggests that first generation immigrants are at a lower risk for a range of health problems and psychopathology than their native-born counterparts, despite sociological disadvantage.[63] The effect has been documented in varied psychological outcomes as well as related outcomes like emotional and sexual abuse of children.[64] Similarly, the Hispanic health paradox refers to an existing literature base showing that, despite exposure to many health risks like low socioeconomic status, limited access to health care and insurance, and reduced education and employment, Hispanics in the U.S. generally report greater health than non-Hispanic Whites.[65] The effect is even more pronounced among Hispanic immigrants; i.e., foreign born.[66]

However, *Serving Refugee Children* depicts the alternate reality of many immigrants—the failure to achieve subjective wellbeing or recuperate psychologically from early adversities. Indeed, empirical research pans out this reality as well. For instance, in some studies, immigrants report higher prevalence of conduct problems, phobias, and early substance use[67]; decreased mental health functioning than their native-born ethnic counterparts[68]; and psychiatric disorder rates comparable to non-Latino White subjects.[69] Critical to *Serving Refugee Children*, accumulating data now indicates that the Hispanic/immigrant advantages cited in previous research do not represent a universal reality and, on the contrary, that certain groups of immigrants, including youth, may be particularly vulnerable to the long term of effects of the psychosocial stressors they encounter.[70] Among others, Luis's story shows the long terms effects of detention during his time and after being released. He clearly lacked adult affection and attached to Lupe and felt apprehensive about moving in with an uncle he had never met before. Lupe still thinks about him and wishes he has adapted well. Generally, this collection clearly reflects a tension apparent in recent empirical literature from the social sciences—tension between the resilience that has typically characterized immigrant adaptation in the U.S. and can motivate an attitude that migrants can and should "pull themselves up by their bootstraps" and the well-documented long-term, handicapping effects of adversity and trauma early in life.

Acculturation, a second framework from the social sciences that emerges in *Serving Refugee Children*, is a bi-dimensional process capturing an individual's connection with their new (post-migration) culture and, separately, connection with their home culture.[71] Individuals high in affiliation with their new culture and low in affiliation with their home culture, for instance, are described as "assimilated," whereas individuals high on both axes are referred to as "bicultural/integrated." Individuals low in both metrics are described as "marginalized" and individuals with high affiliation with their home culture only are referred to as "traditional/separated." Overall, acculturation among immigrants is conceptualized as a change in cultural identity, which includes shifts in various cultural dimensions including typical practices, values, and identifications.[72] Across *Serving Refugee Children*, children's experiences are portrayed at their differing levels of acculturation—some stories show children retaining the games and traditions of their homes and longing for those familiar elements while trying to adapt to life in the U.S. Other narratives show children eager to adopt aspects of U.S. culture, with varying levels of naiveté about it, nonetheless suffering detention and marginalization.

Literature regarding the link between acculturation and mental health is mixed, with some studies of the immigrant paradox reporting that lower acculturation with the host county accounts for health benefits.[73] and others showing that low acculturation among immigrants is risk factor for negative mental health outcomes.[74] *Serving Refugee Children* captures both perspectives—the healing capacity of perceived belonging post-migration and the internal fortitude that comes from affiliation with culture of origin. Indeed, empirical findings do not link simple conceptualizations of high or low acculturation to mental health, rather acculturative stress—self-reported distress during the acculturation process (e.g., distress associated with speaking with an accent)—appears to play a more prominent role in psychological wellbeing after migration.[75]

Relatedly, perceived racism and discrimination—which are featured in *Serving Refugee Children*—have been linked to negative mental health and academic outcomes in immigrant youth in the U.S.[76] Throughout their narratives, children struggle to make sense of their position straddling two countries and cultures, while criminalized or discriminalized. Though the anthology does not explicitly comment on mental health, the impact of this tenuous straddling on children's sense of belonging in the U.S. and longing for there is clearly understood. The emotional bonding of telling stories continues to humanize discussions and immigration policies by fostering a culture of civil rights.

Ultimately, the goal of *Serving Refugee Children* is to bear witness to the children's brave human spirits in their search for safety and their arrival to the U.S. The authors of *Serving Refugee Children* have obscured the identities of the children they serve—changing their names or any other detail that would otherwise identify them in order to cast light on a segment of the immigrant population that has previously been largely excluded from literature and research. No child should have to live the persecution suffered by the majority of unaccompanied immigrant minors, nor should they have to embark upon perilous journeys across Latin America or be subjected to the difficult immigration court process unaided.

Notes

1. "Lupe" is a pseudonym used to protect the identity of the student described.
2. "Enhancing Development Through the Sense of Touch." Urban Child Institute, Urban Child Institute, www.urbanchildinstitute.org/articles/research-to-policy/research/enhancing-development-through-the-sense-of-touch#:~:text=Touch%20not%20only%20impacts%20short,communicate%20their%20needs%20and%20wants
3. For mental health effects on the disruption of migrant youth home environments and use of their first language, see, Jesse Walker, Amanda Venta, and Betsy Galicia. "Who Is Taking Care of Central American Immigrant Youth? Preliminary Data on Caregiving Arrangements and Emotional-Behavioral Symptoms Post-Migration." *Child Psychiatry & Human Development*, 2020; Cassandra Bailey, Emily McIntyre, Aleyda Arreola, and Amanda Venta. "What Are We Missing? How Language Impacts Trauma Narratives," *Journal of Child &Adolescent Trauma* 13 (2020):153–61.
4. Meretoja, Hanna. *The Ethics of Storytelling. Narrative Hermeneutics, History, and the Possible.* New York: Oxford University Press, 2018, 121.
5. Meyers, Diana Tietjens. *Victims' Stories and the Advancement of Human Rights.* New York: Oxford University Press, 2016, 194–95.
6. We have applied the main thesis of Michael P. Nichols's *The Lost Art of Listening* (2009) to the context of listening to undocumented children in immigration detention. Also, see Rubak, Sune, Anneli Sandbæk, Torsten Lauritzen, and Bo Christensen. "Motivational Interviewing: A Systematic Review and Meta-analysis," *British Journal of General Practice* 55, no. 513 (2005): 305–12.
7. Meretoja, 169.
8. Meyers, 16.
9. Ewick, Patricia, and Susan Silbey, "Hegemonic and Subversive Tales: Toward a Sociology of Narrative," *Law & Society Review* 197, no. 29 (1995): 197–226, 219.
10. On the contributions of testimonio, see Alonso, Noemí Acedo. "El género testimonial en Latinoamérica: aproximaciones críticas en busca de su definición, genealogía, y taxonomía," *Latinoamérica. Revista de Estudios Latinoamericanos* 64 (2017): 39–69; Navarrete, Sandra. "Variaciones del testimonio en las ficciones narrativas recientes: diálogos entre Chile y Argentina," *Confluencias* 34.1 (2018): 94–103. For Testimonio Pedagogy, see Ashamawi, Yvonne Pilar El, M. Eugenia Hernández Sánchez, and Judith Flores Carmona, "Testimonialista Pedagogues: Testimonio Pedagogy in Critical Multicultural Education," *International Journal of Multicultural Education* 20.1 (2018): 67–85.
11. Meretoja, 4–5.
12. Meretoja, 141–2.
13. Francesca Polletta. *It Was Like a Fever. Storytelling in Protest and Politics*. Chicago: The University of Chicago Press, 2006, 13.
14. Polletta, 7, 13.
15. Meretoja, 307.
16. Meyers, 188.
17. Meretoja, 109.
18. Polletta, 2.

19. Meyers, 196.
20. Polletta, 19, 24.
21. Ewick and Silbey, 199.
22. Ewick and Silbey, 199.
23. Meyers, 179.
24. Meretoja, 2.
25. Meretoja, 10.
26. Meyers, 178.
27. García Hernández, César Cuauhtémoc . *Migrating to Prison. America's Obsession with Locking up Immigrants.* New York: The New Press, 2019.
28. Bourke, Dale Hanson. *Immigration: Tough Questions, Direct Answers.* Downers Grove: IVP Books, 2014.
29. United Nations High Commission on Refugees. *The State of the World's Refugees,* 2012. Retrieved from: www.unhcr.org/4fcceca9.html
30. Bourke. United Nations General Assembly. *The Refugee Convention, 1951,* 2014. Retrieved from: http://www.unhcr.org/4ca34be29.pdf
31. Bourke (2014).
32. Office of Refugee Resettlement. *Children entering the United States Unaccompanied: Section 1. Placement in ORR Care Provider Facilities,* 2015. Retrieved from: https://www.acf.hhs.gov/orr/resource/children-entering-the-united-states-unaccompanied
33. Office of Refugee Resettlement (2015).
34. Office of Refugee Resettlement (2015).
35. Women's Refugee Commission. *Forced from Home: The Lost boys and Girls of Central America,* 2012. http://www.womensrefugeecomission.org.
36. Furman, Rich et al. "Immigration Detention Centers: Implications for Social Work," *Smith College Studies in Social Work.* 85 (2015), 146–58.
37. Women's Refugee Commission (2012).
38. Chavez-Dueñas, Nayeli, Hector Y. Adames, and Mackenzie T.Goertz. "Esperanza Sin Fronteras: Understanding the Complexities Surrounding the Unaccompanied Refugee Children from Central America," *Latina/o Psychology Today* 10, no. 1 (2014): 10–15.
39. Nayeli et al. (2015).
40. Nayeli et al., (2015).
41. Mark, Michelle. "The Number of Migrant Children in Government Custody Surged to 10,773 under Trump's Policy to Separate Kids from their Parents," *Washington Post,* May 30, 2018.
42. Mark (2018).
43. TRAC (Graph Illustration of Court Data through March 2018). 2018. Juvelines-Immigration Deportation Proceedings. Retrieved from: http://trac.syr.edu/phptools/immigration/juveline
44. U.S. Customs and Border Patrol. *Southwest border unaccompanied alien children (FY2017),* 2017. Retrieved from: https://www.cbp.gov/newsroom/stats/southwest-border-unaccompanied-children/fy-2017.
45. U.S. Customs and Border Patrol. *Southwest border unaccompanied alien children (FY2016),* 2016. Retrieved from: https://www.cbp.gov/newsroom/stats/southwest-border-unaccompanied-children/fy-2016.

46. TRAC (Graph Illustration of Court Data through March 2016). Juvelines-Immigration Deportation Proceedings. 2016. Retrieved from: http://trac.syr.edu/phptools/immigration/juveline

47. Hiskey, Jonathan et al. *Understanding the Central American Refugee Crisis: Why They Are Fleeing and How U.S. Policies Are Failing to Deter Them. American Immigration Council Special Report*. Washington, DC, 2016. Retrieved from: http://immigrationpolicy.org/sites/default/files/docs/understanding_the_central_american_refugee crisis.pdf

48. U.S. Customs and Border Patrol (2016).

49. Venta, Amanda. Letter to the Editor. "The Real Emergency at our Southern Border is Mental Health," *Journal of the American Academy of Child and Adolescent Psychiatry* (June 19, 2019): 1–2; U.S. Conference on Catholic Bishops. *Testimony of Most Reverend Mark Seitz ... On Unaccompanied Children House Judiciary Committee*, 2014. Retrieved from: http://www.usccb.org/about/migration-policy/upload/BSeitzfinaltest.pdf

50. Lesser, Gabriel. and Batalova, Jeanne. Central American Immigrants in the United States. Washington: Migration Policy Institute, 2017. https://www.migrationpolicy.org/article/central-american-immigrants-united-states-4.

51. Masferrer, Claudia, Victor Garcia-Guerrero, and Silvia Giorguli-Saucedo. *Connecting the Dots*. Washington: Migration Policy Institute, 2018. https://www.migrationpolicy.org/article/connecting-dots-emerging-migration-trends-and-policy-questions-north-and-central-america

52. Alvarado, Karina Oliva, Alicia Ivonne Estrada, and Ester E. Hernández (eds.). *US Central Americans: Reconstructing Memories, Struggles, and Communities of Resistance*. Tucson: University of Arizona Press, 2017.

53. Alvarado et al. (2017).

54. Lovato, Roberto. "El Salvador's Gang Violence: The Continuation of Civil War by Other Means," *The Nation* (2015). https://www.thenation.com/article/archive/el-salvadors-gang-violence-continuation-civil-war-other-means/

55. Lovato (2015).

56. Shifter, Michael. *Countering Criminal Violence in Central America* (No. 64). Council on Foreign Relations, 2012. https://cdn.cfr.org/sites/default/files/pdf/2012/03/Criminal_Violence_CSR64.pdf?_ga=2.100644830.1318443129.1581026443-1004628872.1581026443

57. Shifter (2012).

58. Martinez, Sofía. "Today's Migrant Flow is Different," *The Atlantic* (2018). https://www.theatlantic.com/international/archive/2018/06/central-america-border-immigration/563744/

59. Shifter (2012)

60. Vogt, Wendy. *Lives in Transit: Violence and Intimacy on the Migrant Journey*. Ockland: University of California Press, 2018, 139–65, 209.

61. Fores Tamayo has previously published this poem in Democracy Chronicles (https://democracychronicles.org/new-poetry-elegy-to-a-refugee-girl/); Adjunct Justice (https://adjunct-justice.blogspot.com/2018/06/elegy-to-refugee-girloda-una-nina.html). In Literary Yard https://literaryyard.com/2019/07/25/las-azucenas-and-other-poems-by-ana-m-fores-tamayo/ and in *What Rough Beast*, Indolent Books https://www.indolentbooks.com/what-rough-beast-poem-for-september-24-2019/

62. See Freedom for Immigrants report on how immigration detention has been portrayed in the media since 2009. https://www.dropbox.com/s/p2mov8td2dkl6nb/CIVIC_ImmigrationDetention_Media_Final.pdf?dl=0

63. Lui, Priscilla P. "Intergenerational Cultural Conflict, Mental Health, and Educational Outcomes Among Asian and Latino/a Americans: Qualitative and Meta-analytic Review," *Psychological Bulletin*, 141, no. 2 (2015): 404; Wolff, Kevin T. et al. "The Protective Impact of Immigrant Concentration on Juvenile Recidivism: A Statewide Analysis of Youth Offenders," *Journal of Criminal Justice*, 43, no. 6 (2015): 522–31; MacDonald, John, and Jessica Saunders. "Are Immigrant Youth Less Violent? Specifying the Reasons and Mechanisms," *The Annals of the American Academy of Political and Social Science* 641, no. 1 (2012): 125–47; Acevedo-Garcia, Dolores, and Lisa M. Bates. "Latino Health Paradoxes: Empirical Evidence, Explanations, Future Research, and Implications." In *Latinas/os in the United States: Changing the Face of America*. Eds. Rodriguez, Havidan, Saenz, Rogelio, Menjivar, Cecilia (Eds.) New York: Springer, 2008, 101–13; Vaughn, M. G., C. P. Salas-Wright, M. DeLisi, and B. R. Maynard. "The Immigrant Paradox: Immigrants Are Less Antisocial than Native-Born Americans," *Social Psychiatry and Psychiatric Epidemiology* 49, no. 7 (2014): 1129–37.

64. Millett, Kate. *Sexual Politics*. New York: Columbia University Press, 1970, 2016.

65. Ruiz, John M. et al. "The Hispanic Health Paradox: From Epidemiological Phenomenon to Contribution Opportunities for Psychological Science," *Group Processes & Intergroup Relations* 19, n. 4 (2016), 462–76.

66. Singh, Gopal K., Alfonso Rodriguez-Lainz, and Michael D. Kogan. "Immigrant Health Inequalities in the United States: Use of Eight Major National Data Systems." *The Scientific World Journal* (2013).

67. Breslau, Joshua et al. "Health Selection among Migrants from Mexico to the US: Childhood Predictors of Adult Physical and Mental Health." *Public Health Reports*, 2011, 361–70.

68. Farley, Tillman et al. "Stress, Coping, and Health: A Comparison of Mexican immigrants, Mexican-Americans, and Non-Hispanic Whites," *Journal of Immigrant Health* 7, n. 3 (2005): 213–20.

69. Alegría, Margarita et al. "Prevalence of Mental Illness in Immigrant and Non-immigrant US Latino Groups," *American Journal of Psychiatry* 165, n. 3 (2008): 359–69.

70. Teruya, Stacey A. and Shahrzad Bazargan-Hejazi, "The Immigrant and Hispanic Paradoxes a Systematic Review of their Predictions and Effects," *Hispanic Journal of Behavioral Sciences* 35, n. 4 (2013): 486–509.

71. Sam, David L., and John W. Berry, "Acculturation When Individuals and Groups of Different Cultural Backgrounds Meet." *Perspectives on Psychological Science* 5, n. 4 (2010): 472–81.

72. Schwartz, Seth J. et al. "Rethinking the Concept of Acculturation: Implications for Theory and Research," *American Psychologist*, 65 (2010): 237–51.

73. Kaplan, Mark S., and Gary Marks. "Adverse Effects of Acculturation: Psychological Distress Among Mexican American Young Adults," *Social Science & Medicine* 31, n. 12 (1990): 1313–19.

74. Hwang, Wei-Chin., and Julia Y. Ting, "Disaggregating the Effects of Acculturation and Acculturative Stress on the Mental Health of Asian Americans," *Cultural Diversity and Ethnic Minority Psychology* 14, n. 2 (2008): 147–54.

75. Caplan, Susan. "Latinos, Acculturation, and Acculturative Stress: A Dimensional Concept Analysis." *Policy, Politics, & Nursing Practice*, 8, n. 2 (2007): 93–106; Turner, R. Jay; Donald A. Lloyd, and John Taylor. "Stress Burden, Drug Dependence and the Nativity Paradox among US Hispanics," *Drug and Alcohol Dependence* 83, n. 1 (2006), 79–89; Teruya, S. A., and S. Bazargan-Hejazi. "The Immigrant and Hispanic Paradoxes a Systematic Review of their Predictions and Effects," *Hispanic Journal of Behavioral Sciences* 35, n. 4, (2013): 486–509.

76. Suárez-Orozco, Carola; Jean Rhodes, and Michael Milburn. "Unraveling the Immigrant Paradox: Academic Engagement and Disengagement Among Recently Arrived Immigrant Youth," *Youth and Society* 41, n. 2 (2009): 151–85; Smokowski, Paul R., and Martica L. Bacallao. "Acculturation and Aggression in Latino Adolescents: A Structural Model Focusing on Cultural Risk Factors and Assets," *Journal of Abnormal Child Psychology* 34, n. 5 (2006), 657–71.

References

Acedo Alonso, Noemí. "El género testimonial en Latinoamérica: aproximaciones críticas en busca de su definición, genealogía, y taxonomía," *Latinoamérica. Revista de Estudios Latinoamericanos* 64 (2017): 39–69.

Acevedo-Garcia, Dolores, and Bates, Lisa M. "Latino Health Paradoxes: Empirical Evidence, Explanations, Future Research, and Implications." In *Latinas/os in the United States: Changing the Face of America*, 101–113. New York: Springer, 2008.

Alegría, Margarita et al. "Prevalence of Mental Illness in Immigrant and Non-immigrant US Latino Groups." *American Journal of Psychiatry*. 165, n. 3 (2008): 359–69.

Alvarado, Karina Oliva, Alicia Ivonne Estrada, and Ester E. Hernández (eds.). *US Central Americans: Reconstructing Memories, Struggles, and Communities of Resistance*. Tucson: University of Arizona Press, 2017.

Anzaldúa, Gloria. *Friends from the Other Side/Amigos del otro lado*. San Francisco: Children's Book Press, 1993.

Argueta, Jorge. *We Are Like the Clouds/Somos como las nubes*. Toronto: Groundwood Books, 2016.

Bourke, Dale Hanson. *Immigration: Tough Questions, Direct Answers*. Downers Grove: IVP Books, 2014.

Breslau, Joshua et al. *Health Selection among Migrants from Mexico to the US: Childhood Predictors of Adult Physical and Mental Health*. Public Health Reports, 2011, 361–70.

Buitrago, Jairo. *Two White Rabbits*. Toronto: Groundwood Books, 2015.

Caplan, Susan. "Latinos, Acculturation, and Acculturative Stress: A Dimensional Concept Analysis," *Policy, Politics, & Nursing Practice*, 8, n. 2 (2007): 93–106.

Chavez-Dueñas, Nayeli, Hector Y. Adames, and Mackenzie T. Goertz. "Esperanza Sin Fronteras: Understanding the Complexities Surrounding the Unaccompanied Refugee Children from Central America," *Latina/o Psychology Today* 10, n. 1 (2014): 10–15.

Cisneros, Sandra. *The House of Mango Street*. New York: Vintage Books, 1984.

Colato Laínez, René. *From North to South/Del Norte al Sur*. San Francisco: Children's Book Press, 2010.

Colato Laínez, René. *Waiting for Papá. Esperando a Papá*. Houston: Piñata Books, 2004.

Danticat, Edwidge. *Mama's Nightingale: A Story of Immigration and Separation*. New York: Dial Books, 2015.

El Ashamawi, Yvonne Pilar, M. Eugenia Hernández Sánchez, and Judith Flores Carmona. "Testimonialista Pedagogues: Testimonio Pedagogy in Critical Multicultural Education," *International Journal of Multicultural Education* 20, n. 1 (2018): 67–85.

Farley, Tillman et al. "Stress, Coping, and Health: A Comparison of Mexican immigrants, Mexican-Americans, and Non-Hispanic Whites," *Journal of Immigrant Health* 7, n. 3 (2005): 213–20.

Furman, Rich et al. "Immigration Detention Centers: Implications for Social Work," *Smith College Studies in Social Work* 85 (2015): 146–58.

Hiskey, Jonathan et al. *Understanding the Central American Refugee Crisis: Why They Are Fleeing and How U.S. Policies Are Failing to Deter Them*. American Immigration Council Special Report. Washington, DC, 2016. Retrieved from: http://immigrationpolicy.org/sites/default/files/docs/understanding_the_central_american_refugee_crisis.pdf

Hwang, Wei-Chin., and Julia Y. Ting. "Disaggregating the Effects of Acculturation and Acculturative Stress on the Mental Health of Asian Americans," *Cultural Diversity and Ethnic Minority Psychology* 14, n. 2 (2008): 147–54.

Jiménez, Francisco. *The Circuit: Stories from the Life of a Migrant Child*. Albuquerque: University of New Mexico Press, 1997.

Jiménez, Francisco. *Breaking Through*. Boston: HMH Books for Young Readers, 2001.Kaplan, Mark S., and Gary Marks. "Adverse Effects of Acculturation: Psychological Distress Among Mexican American Young Adults," *Social Science & Medicine* 31, n. 12 (1990): 1313–19.

Kim, Patti. *Here I Am*. Minnesota: Capstone, 2013.

Lesser, Gabriel, and Jeanne Batalova. Central American Immigrants in the United States. Washington: Migration Policy Institute, 2017. https://www.migrationpolicy.org/article/central-american-immigrants-united-states-4

Lovato, Roberto. "El Salvador's Gang Violence: The Continuation of Civil War By Other Means," *The Nation* (2015). https://www.thenation.com/article/archive/el-salvadors-gang-violence-continuation-civil-war-other-means/

Lui, Priscilla P. "Intergenerational Cultural Conflict, Mental Health, and Educational Outcomes Among Asian and Latino/a Americans: Qualitative and Meta-analytic Review," *Psychological Bulletin* 141, n. 2 (2015): 404.

MacDonald, John, and Jessica Saunders. "Are Immigrant Youth Less Violent? Specifying the Reasons and Mechanisms," *The Annals of the American Academy of Political and Social Science* 641, n. 1 (2012): 125–47.

Mark, Michelle. "The Number of Migrant Children in Government Custody Surged to 10,773 under Trump's Policy to Separate Kids from their Parents." *Washington Post*, May 30, 2018.

Martinez, Sofía. "Today's Migrant Flow is Different." *The Atlantic* (2018). https://www.theatlantic.com/international/archive/2018/06/central-america-border-immigration/563744/

Masferrer, Claudia, Victor Garcia-Guerrero, and Silvia Giorguli-Saucedo. Connecting the Dots. Washington: Migration Policy Institute, 2018. https://www.migrationpolicy.org/article/connecting-dots-emerging-migration-trends-and-policy-questions-north-and-central-america

Mateo, José Manuel. *Migrant: The Journey of a Mexican Worker.* New York: Abrams Books, 2014.

Meretoja, Hanna. *The Ethics of Storytelling. Narrative Hermeneutics, History, and the Possible.* New York: Oxford University Press, 2018.

Michelson, Seth. *Dreaming America.* Silver Spring: Settlement House, 2017.

Millett, Kate. *Sexual Politics.* New York: Columbia University Press, 1970, 2016.

Navarrete, Sandra. "Variaciones del testimonio en las ficciones narrativas recientes: diálogos entre Chile y Argentina," *Confluencias* 34, n. 1 (2018): 94–103.

Nazario, Sonia. *Enrique's Journey: The Story of a Boy's Dangerous Odyssey to Reunite with His Mother.* New York: Random House, 2007.

Office of Refugee Resettlement. *Children entering the United States Unaccompanied: Section 1. Placement in ORR Care Provider Facilities.* 2015. Retrieved from: https://www.acf.hhs.gov/orr/resource/children-entering-the-united-states-unaccompanied

Resau, Laura. *Star in the Forest.* New York: Yearling Books, 2012.

Rivera, Tomás. *. . . y no se lo tragó la tierra.* Houston: Arte Público Press, 1988.

Rubak, Sune, Anneli Sandbæk, Torsten Lauritzen, and Bo Christensen . "Motivational Interviewing: A Systematic Review and Meta-Analysis," *British Journal of General Practice* 55, no. 513 (2005): 305–12.

Ruiz, John M. et al. "The Hispanic Health Paradox: From Epidemiological Phenomenon to Contribution Opportunities for Psychological Science," *Group Processes & Intergroup Relations* 19, n. 4 (2016): 462–76.

Sam, David L., and Berry, John W. "Acculturation When Individuals and Groups of Different Cultural Backgrounds Meet." *Perspectives on Psychological Science* 5 (4) (2010), 472–81.

Schwartz, Seth J. et al. "Rethinking the Concept of Acculturation: Implications for Theory and Research." *American Psychologist* 65 (2010): 237–51.

Shifter, Michael. *Countering Criminal Violence in Central America* (No. 64). Council on Foreign Relations, 2012. https://cdn.cfr.org/sites/default/files/pdf/2012/03/Criminal_Violence_CSR64.pdf?_ga=2.100644830.1318443129.1581026443–1004628872.1581026443

Singh, Gopal K., Alfonso Rodriguez-Lainz, and Michael D. Kogan. "Immigrant Health Inequalities in the United States: Use of Eight Major National Data Systems," *The Scientific World Journal* (2013). https://www.hindawi.com/journals/tswj/2013/512313/

Smokowski, Paul R., and Martica L. Bacallao. "Acculturation and Aggression in Latino Adolescents: A Structural Model Focusing on Cultural Risk Factors and Assets." *Journal of Abnormal Child Psychology* 34, n. 5 (2006): 657–71.

Suárez-Orozco, Carola, Jean Rhodes, and Michael Milburn. "Unraveling the Immigrant Paradox: Academic Engagement and Disengagement Among Recently Arrived Immigrant Youth." *Youth and Society* 41, n. 2 (2009): 151–85.

Terrio, Susan J. *Whose Child Am I?: Unaccompanied, Undocumented Children in U.S. Immigration Custody.* Berkeley: University of California Press, 2015.

Teruya, Stacey A., and Shahrzad Bazargan-Hejazi. "The Immigrant and Hispanic Paradoxes a Systematic Review of their Predictions and Effects." *Hispanic Journal of Behavioral Sciences*, 35, n. 4 (2013): 486–509.

TRAC (Graph Illustration of Court Data through March 2016). Juvelines-Immigration Deportation Proceedings. 2016. Retrieved from: http://trac.syr.edu/phptools/immigration/juveline

TRAC (Graph Illustration of Court Data through March 2018). Juvelines-Immigration Deportation Proceedings. 2018. Retrieved from: http:// trac.syr.edu/phptools/immigration/juveline

Turner, R. Jay, Donald A. Lloyd, and John Taylor. "Stress Burden, Drug Dependence and the Nativity Paradox among US Hispanics," *Drug and Alcohol Dependence* 83, n. 1 (2006), 79–89.

U.S. Conference on Catholic Bishops. *Testimony of Most Reverend Mark Seitz . . . On Unaccompanied Children House Judiciary Committee*, 2014. Retrieved from: http://www.usccb.org/about/migration-policy/upload/BSeitzfinaltest.pdf

U.S. Customs and Border Patrol. *Southwest Border Unaccompanied Alien Children (FY2016)*, 2016. Retrieved from: https://www.cbp.gov/newsroom/stats/southwest-border-unaccompanied-children/fy-2016.

U.S. Homeland Security. *Public Law 107–296*, 2002. Retrieved from: https://www.dhs.gov/sites/default/files/publications/hr_5005_enr.pdf

United Nations General Assembly. *The Refugee Convention, 1951*. Retrieved from: http://www.unhcr.org/4ca34be29.pdf

United Nations High Commission on Refugees. *The State of the World's Refugees*, 2012. Retrieved from: www.unhcr.org/4fcceca9.html

Vaughn, Michael G., Christopher P. Salas-Wright, Matt DeLisi, and Brandy R. Maynard. "The Immigrant Paradox: Immigrants Are Less Antisocial than Native-Born Americans," *Social Psychiatry and Psychiatric Epidemiology* 49, n. 7 (2014): 1129–1137.

Venta, Amanda. Letter to the Editor. "The Real Emergency at our Southern Border is Mental Health." *Journal of the American Academy of Child and Adolescent Psychiatry*, (June 19, 2019): 1–2.

Wolff, Kevin T. et al. "The Protective Impact of Immigrant Concentration on Juvenile Recidivism: A Statewide Analysis of Youth Offenders." *Journal of Criminal Justice*, 43, n. 6 (2015): 522–531.

Women's Refugee Commission. *Forced from Home: The Lost boys and Girls of Central America*. 2012. http://www.womensrefugeecomission.org

Part I
ESCAPES AND CROSSINGS

· 1 ·

SETH MICHELSON

For the past few years Michelson has had the honor of working with and for undocumented, unaccompanied youth (13 to 17 years of age) in one of the two maximum-security detention centers in the East Coast. More specifically, in that detention center, Michelson has led weekly poetry workshops with the children, and from that collaboration he has edited and translated their writing to create the anthology *Dreaming America: Voices of Undocumented Youth in Maximum-Security Detention*. Seth Michelson particularly remembers the harrowing story of Luz, an undocumented, unaccompanied minor he recently met during a poetry workshop. Her story of migration from El Salvador to incarceration in the United States shows her courage, determination, hope, and indomitable spirit.

Looking for Luz

That morning at the poetry workshop Luz told me that she could hardly believe her good luck: Abuela had given her ten dollars to buy chicken, saying she could buy herself lipstick with any change. And change there would be. In her bubbly excitement that summer morning, Luz rushed out of their one-bedroom apartment in Soyapango, San Salvador, already knowing exactly what color lipstick she wanted. It was a shade of red, carmine red, deep and lustrous as a sun-kissed jocote, the same color that Susana, the most popular girl in school, had debuted just last week, making it all the rage among the girls in their ninth-grade class at Escuela Panamericana.

"Hurry back, Luz," Abuela had told her, ushering the teen out the door with a loving pat on the bottom, this treasured grandchild, Abuela's only one, and so she spoiled the child, as with the lipstick. *Se lo merece*, Abuela thought, watching Luz bounce away. *Es tan dulce, tan buena. Gracias, Dios, por esta gran bendición.*

And with that Abuela tuned back to the kitchen to resume prepping the family's weekly Sunday lunch in her apartment, where she lived with Luz and her mother, and where Abuela's other two children, Luz's tios, would soon arrive, too, to eat with them.

They were a small but happy family, tightknit and tender, a rarity anywhere in the world, and especially here in this neighborhood rife with gangs and drug-addicts and abusive police constantly running people off or sending them to prison, breaking up families.

Against such rupture, Luz's family seemed in fact set to grow: Just this morning Tío Marcos and Tío Edilber had each called Abuela to ask if they could bring their new girlfriends to lunch, too, an auspicious omen.

"*Claro, m'ijo*," she'd replied to each of them with joy in her voice. "*Siempre hay lugar.* There's a place for everyone."

Hence the last-minute need for more chicken, and Abuela knew Luz was good for it. She was smart and quick as a rabbit, both at home and in school. *Ay, tesoro mío*, thought Abuela, smiling while kneading masa for pupusas.

Meanwhile Luz was already outside, bounding up the street towards the Super Selecto market, her jet-black braids bouncing against her back like happy seals doing flips and twirls. She was thinking about the lipstick while fingering the velvety bill in her purse, slung diagonally across her chest for added security.

As she hustled along, the morning light was so bright it made her squint, causing her to realize she'd forgotten her sunglasses in her hurry.

"Shoot," she thought. "A double blow." She'd not only have to endure the harsh glare of light with her naked eyes, but also walk in public without having the glasses to break up the long oval of her face. It was a beauty trick she'd learned two months back from an article in a women's magazine—"Fashion Tips for Summer 2016"—and she'd practiced it religiously ever since, having long worried with typical teen insecurity that her face was hideous, monstrously huge and fleshy, her ugliest feature.

Looking down to avoid the light and to hide her face, Luz pushed on, feeling self-conscious, conspicuous, but by now a mere three blocks from the Super Selecto. "So close! *¡Casi llego!*" And she hoped she wouldn't see anyone she knew and have to stop and make small talk, when all she wanted to do was lose herself in the make-up aisle. "*¿Mágico o rojo místico?*" she was wondering, already shopping in her head, as the soft hem of her flowery skirt whipped behind her in a tailwind, marking her speed and purpose.

And like that, lost in thought, hurrying along while looking downward, she almost bumped into someone coming straight at her on the sidewalk. Kelvin. "*Uh oh.*"

"*Mira, chica,* watch where you are going," he said bluntly but with a smile, one silver incisor glinting.

"*Perdón,*" Luz muttered through an embarrassed grimace, looking down again.

She attempted to sidestep Kelvin and continue on her journey, but he sidestepped, too, mirroring her body. He then grabbed her shoulders roughly in his hands, and looked her up and down, leering.

"Daaaamn, girl," he said. "You lookin' good. All grown and shit."

Luz shuddered. Kelvin led the local clica of MS-13. Everyone knew to avoid him.

He'd spent three years in prison, where it was rumored, he'd killed two people, and he was always out here robbing and beating and bullying and licking his lips.

Luz wanted to get away, and quickly, but his grip on her shoulders was firm.

"*¿Qué te pasa, Luz?*" he asked.

The question made her feel like there was a rockslide behind her ribs.

"You afraid of me, girl?" he asked, tonguing his silver incisor. "Well don't be! I'll treat you good."

"*Es que tengo prisa,*" she answered quickly, trying again to free herself, get around him. But he held on, and in the burning light, his bald head looked to her like it was wreathed in flames.

He began to swivel his head, looking long and hard up and down the block. Luz watched the skull tattoo on his neck stretch and compress as he moved, as if it were some sort of ghostly minion helping him.

Quick as a viper's strike, Kelvin clapped a hand over Luz's unpainted lips and dragged her into the adjacent alley, abandoned but for a plastic bag tumbling away in a soft breeze.

Luz's eyes bulged with fear. She felt frozen, could hardly breathe.

"Yeah, you lookin' good, girl," he was murmuring as he dragged her behind a dumpster, one hand still muzzling her mouth, the other tracing its way up her thigh and under her skirt, till he screamed out in pain.

"Bitch, why you bite me?" he boomed, his dark eyes compressed to vicious slits, as he shook and waved a bloody hand about in the air, furious, hopping in place. "Bitch, I'm gonna kill you!"

With his good hand, he pulled a pistol from his waistband, and Luz, finally able to move, turned to run, before falling in place, two bullets in her head.

***

"*M'ija,* you have to go," Luz's mother was saying through tears. "You have to go North, to the United States. It's the only way, *m'ija.* Please."

"*No puedo, Mamá,*" Luz was sobbing. "I won't go. I can't do it."

Her mother pulled her into a soft embrace, and the two sobbed and sobbed, standing there, smack in the middle of Abuela's living room.

Mamá sobbed and sobbed with the thought of losing her only child, her precious Luz.

Luz sobbed and sobbed even though her head throbbed with incandescent pain. It felt as if someone were driving a metal spike on fire into her left ear and out her face through her nose. And the pain in her heart was worse.

She sobbed and sobbed, having been home from the hospital less than a day after a week of emergency surgeries that had saved her life after the shooting.

She sobbed and sobbed, though she was still deaf in one ear and a high-pitched ringing filled her head incessantly, not to mention the dizziness, nausea, sudden bouts of vomiting.

She'd been like this for days, but the doctors had insisted she was ready to go home. Had said over and over to her in the hospital how lucky she'd been. "*Has tenido mucha suerte, Luz,*" they'd say. "You're a very lucky girl." And then they'd stand there smiling at her, self-satisfied, as if they'd fixed everything.

At first, she'd believed them, despite a constant pain that sometimes surged so strongly it would blind her temporarily, like a massive bolt of lightning, the agony literally knocking her to her knees. "A very lucky girl." Still they'd insisted.

"A clean through-and-though," they'd called it, showing her x-rays of where the first bullet had entered her head behind her left ear and then exited her left nostril. "The best possible outcome considering the placement. Of times a bullet will rattle around in there and do all sorts of damage."

They'd marvel, too, at the second bullet: how it had miraculously been even less intrusive, less damaging, how it had lodged itself between her scalp and skull at the crown of her head, stopped dead in its tracks, so to speak, before being able to rip into her brain.

"Ay, *m'ija*," her mother was cooing, "*Ya lo sé*. I know, I know." Her hushed voice sounded thin, wounded, distant.

"If Kelvin finds out you survived," Abuela chimed in, "he'll come back to kill you, *m'ija*. It's no joke, and it's no discussion. You have to go. You're going."

Behind the surgical mask covering her disfigured nose, Luz felt like she was disappearing, crumbling inward. Her heavily bandaged head shook above her frail body, which quaked with fear. She couldn't go, wouldn't go. I just wasn't possible. She didn't even want to leave her mother's embrace, let alone this apartment, the fold-out couch she shared with her mother since birth, the only home she'd known. And now she had to leave it, leave Soyapango, leave El Salvador?

"I can't," she sobbed. "*No puedo, Mamá*. I can't do it."

But she knew, too, that she had to or she'd be killed by Kelvin or one of his minions.

***

The entire family—Abuela, Mamá, Tío Marcos, Tío Edilber, and Luz—gathered morosely at the dinner table that evening to pool together their money for her journey to the United States.

"Four hundred and fifty-three dollars?" Tío Edilber was asking as he finished counting it all. "That all we got?" He shook his head. They all fell silent, knowing it insufficient. Even if riding La Bestia for free across Mexico, Luz would still need at least a thousand dollars to be minimally comfortable and safe. But this was all they had, and she had to go. There were already rumors of Kelvin having heard about her survival.

No one spoke. Abuela stroked Luz's back as the child wept silently at her side.

"Listen, Luz," Tío Marcos said, feigning smile in his voice. "When you get to gringolandia, they'll fix you up good. They have the best doctors in the world. They'll make you look like Shakira if you want to!"

But his gentle gesture fell flat, and his voice dissolved into the heaviness of the room like a pinch of sugar dissolving into dark black tea.

"Tomorrow morning, *m'ija*," Mamá was saying. "It's because I love you. It's because we love you. And because you're stronger than you know."

***

The next morning at 7am, Luz, wearing a pink backpack with an apple, a banana, and a bottle of water in it, boarded the bus in the Terminal de Occidente.

The ticket had cost her $36, blowing a hole through her budget, but nowhere near as big the hole in her heart through which she was free-falling, spiraling down in a seemingly bottomless pit, which rang with the same shrill noise that had continuously filled her head since surgery, like a soundtrack to her life since the shooting.

Luz climbed into the bus and took her seat as if outside of her body watching herself do it. She felt hollow, weightless, a swirl of confusion, loneliness, and fear. The admixture coursed through her, making her tremble. She felt like she was trapped in an icy shower. Her head throbbed as usual with the pulsating pain, and she barely noticed the tears running down her cheeks and into the surgical mask hiding her disfigured nose.

As the engine of the bus roared to life, she couldn't bear to look out the window at her family, gathered on the curb just on the other side of her window to wave goodbye to her. Instead, she looked down at her lap and watched teardrops explode on her knees as if in slow-motion. Her hands trembled so much that she decided to sit on them, and in that pose, she began to roll away.

Alone in her window seat, she looked so tiny, so vulnerable, a small child drowning dead center in a massive lake, unreachable.

She longed to be again on Abuela's lumpy sofa, laughing at *novelas* with her.

"How will I survive without her? without Mamá? Without *mis tíos*? When will I see them next?"

The bus bumped and belched its way out of the station, the first of many in a zigzagging three-day series of stops that would hopefully carry Luz safely to Tapachula, Chiapas.

***

It was pitch black out and freezing cold when Luz awoke. *Have I lost my vision?* she wondered, seeing nothing at first until the world slowly returned to her, a darkness unfolding.

Her surgical mask was stuck to her shattered nose by dried blood, and it hurt to adjust it. Her head throbbed with the usual pain, and it was filled with the customary harsh ringing, that pain and the noise her only two companions on this journey, the only things familiar, predictable, known.

"*Dios mío*," she whispered. "I can't do this. I'm not strong enough. God, take me here."

Luz had no idea where she was or what time it was or what she would do if God indeed forced her to live this nightmarish pre-dawn. And she was hungry. She was tired. She was scared and alone and in physical agony.

Luz wanted to give in, to quit this impossible journey, to be revoked by God from Earth to the heavens, the dark sky all around her engulfing her, swallowing her into sweet oblivion.

Just then an old Guatemalan woman's warm hand slipped itself into Luz's, interlocking their fingers. The old woman, as if by magic, then lifted Luz from her seat and into the aisle with her.

Standing there in the silent darkness, they locked eyes. Luz saw a radiant kindness in the old woman's pupils; the old woman saw Luz's pain. It was as obvious as it was common in children traveling this route, especially when alone, and over the past few years, the old woman had seen it in the eyes of thousands of migrating youth: guatemaltecos, hondureños, salvadoreños, nicaragüenses—all of them passing through her home state of San Marcos, which she herself traversed daily, selling homemade tamales from a plastic basket wrapped in a blanket to eke out her living bus stop by bus stop.

"Come with me, *m'ija*," she said gently, careful not to frighten the girl with noise.

Wrapped in layers of sweaters and a faded scarf, the old woman led Luz off the bus in Melacatán, the las stop in Guatemala, desolate in this pre-dawn lull but for a few bus drivers smoking cigarettes and a scattering of sleepy passengers milling about the station in these final, chilly hours before daybreak to keep warm.

She pressed a hot tamale into Luz's hand, and the sudden warmth spread through Luz's fingers, which, stiff and clenched with cold, began to loosen, opening the way an orchid unfurls in humid heat. The warmth radiated up Luz's arm and into her chest, where it lodged itself like a tiny sunrise, a new-found star deep within her body, a tiny hope rekindled.

"If you don't have papers, *mi amor*," whispered the old woman to Luz, petting her hand, "then it's best to walk up the block and around that building over there, see? Just beyond it, there's an alley. Follow it until it opens into a field, cross over the culvert, and you'll find yourself in a dry riverbed. If you can cross it in the dark, you'll avoid being seen. You may even see others there doing the same. Don't be afraid. Just keep moving."

She was whispering so softly now that Luz could hardly hear her, even when turning her one good ear directly to the old lady's lips and leaning in close.

"You're *my angel, mi vida*," she thought she heard the old woman say in conclusion.

But Luz knew, too, how disorientated she felt, how sick with pain. Her face throbbed, her head was ringing, and she was cold and numb with fear. And she was hungry, she was thirsty, and she needed to pee. So, she simply nodded and whispered, "*Gracias, Señora*."

"Ok," said the old woman. "*Ten cuidado*. Be careful, *m'ija*. There are thieves everywhere, even ones with badges and truncheons. Go now, *m'ija*. Be quick and invisible."

And Luz went.

***

When recalling her 1,450-mile trip from Tapachula to Monterrey on top of La Bestia, the Train of the Dead, all Luz could recall was the anguish. For 1,450 miles she bounced on the roof of cargo cars, shoulder to shoulder with other seated people, rain and wind and sun punishing them, exposed night and day, though nights were often far worse because of the vicious chill, whether in forest, jungle, or desert. It was the way the sun would drop like a failed lottery ticket, another lost opportunity to see the world anew, another day of soot and hunger and exposure turning to the dark desolation of a night to shiver through with all the other exhausted dreamers were slowly dehydrating, losing hope and energy.

Yes, nights had definitely been the worst: hour after hour felt like bathing in ice water under a strong fan that never stopped blowing. It felt like having icicles shaped into swords and thrust through your chest and throat over and over. And if ever she slept, she'd often wake to being fondled in the pitch black by wheezing men—her breasts, thighs, and bottom groped and pinched and pawed at and pinched. Once she'd even woken to hot, sticky lips moving up and down the side of her neck like slugs. And each time it happened, she'd go stiff with terror, unable to cry out, let alone flee. Luz mute as a statue. Luz punished by this looping abuse as they rattled northward.

Worse, she'd see Kelvin's face mapped over each and every molesters'. Kelvin snarling at her with that silver tooth. Kelvin's hand under her skirt. The bang of two quick gunshots, the waking to pain in hospital, the queasy stinging when she'd have to peel surgical masks from her face, where dried blood had crusted them to her shattered nose.

Plus, there was the hunger on La Bestia. Hunger like she'd never known. A sucking hole in her belly into which it felt like her whole being was constantly being pulled into, hunger of oblivion, of endless tornado, of the atomization of the will to live.

And she could do nothing. On her first day atop the train, she'd bought two bags of chips, which left her thirsty. So, an hour later, when she saw a boy appear atop their car hawking soda and water, she bought a bagful of orange Fanta. But instead of soda, he'd pulled out a machete and demanded her entire purse, which he promptly ran off with. Others knew of the boy, a local mara, but no one had warned Luz.

Towards the end of the journey, whenever the train would stop, she'd climb down and forage for garbage to eat, and if unable to find any, she'd pull and chew grass like a runaway goat, feeling a shame so deep and thorough that she wondered aloud if she were still human.

***

When Luz finally hopped off La Bestia for the last time, she was just outside of Monterrey, Nuevo León, leaving her about 200 miles to reach Laredo, Texas, the famed *Estados Unidos*, Land of the Free.

But Luz wasn't sure she could do it. She was exhausted, filthy, penniless, famished, and desperately lonely. Her head still pounded with pain that felt like a bomb exploding again and again from her nose. And she was still deaf in one ear, changing her relation to the outside world, and inside her skull, the usual piercing buzz scuttled any attempt to organize her thoughts, calm her nerves.

She began to scratch her forearms beneath her filthy clothes that had made her skin dry and itchy. And her scalp itched, too, beneath hair thick and matted with grease and dirt and dried sweat, though she dared not scratch it for fear of dislodging the scabs over her bullet holes and beginning to bleed again, this time with nothing on hand to try to staunch it.

Like this, she wandered away from the bus, feeling hideous, monstrous, abandoned by humanity, God, Jesus, and the Virgin of Guadalupe. She abandoned the plan that Tío Marcos had outlined for her, which at this point had called for her to hitchhike up the 85 Highway to the border, maybe even making across in the vehicle if fortunate enough to luck into a Chicano family with papers traveling back to the US and blending in with them, gliding through a checkpoint with a practiced smile of shy innocence.

But no. That was a plan for a different Luz, from a different era she could hardly remember. So instead of heading for the highway, Luz veered off course, headed into the nearby desert, desolate but for creosote, cactus, and a lone buzzard circling in the distance.

Meanwhile her fellow travelers from the bus set off northbound in clusters to seek their destinies. Luz heard them go, knew the right direction, but she just couldn't muster the strength to follow, to hope.

After meandering for about a hundred yards, she flopped down in the sand behind an ancient saguaro, her courage as depleted as her stamina after so many days of hunger, abuse, and punishing loneliness.

Racked with pain and anguish, exhausted, she put a handful of sand into her mouth and chewed, hoping it would help her to dissolve into the desert, slip away in a peaceful death right now, right here, transporting her spirit someplace where her head wouldn't hurt and where she couldn't be groped, robbed, or beaten.

Still chewing slowly, she zipped up her hoodie until it left but a small hole, and she began to pray to be engulfed. And while she waited to be taken, she concentrated on the pulsating pain emanating from the bullet holes in her head, her shattered nose. And she began to cry, a deep, shaking grief, which surprised her with the violence of its spasming the way sudden thunder sometimes shakes the sky and then comes the explosive, raging downpour.

***

Who knows how long Luz had been huddled there, sobbing alone in the desert, when again an old woman appeared. This time it was *Abuela*.

"¡*Abuela!*" Luz cried out, coming to her senses.

She scrambled up from the ground, a big smile on her face behind her tattered surgical mask, streaked with dried blood.

The two shared a deep and warm embrace, Luz burying her face into *Abuela's* neck and saying "*Abuela*, so good to see you! Thank you for coming!"

Then the old woman pulled away.

"*M'ija*," she said softly. "I'm not your abuela. My name is Alicia Benitez Rodríguez. I'm Mexican, from here."

Luz was confused. She'd heard the words, had even noticed the odd Mexican accent with which Abuela was speaking, but she was sure it was *Abuela* standing there, it was *Abuela*'s face, she'd recognize her sparkling eyes anywhere, her ruddy cheeks.

"Are you alright, *m'ija?*" the old woman asked, a shawl over her head, making her look like some kind of wandering desert *Santa Abuela*.

Luz said nothing, just stared into that familiar loving face. She was still so confused by the strange voice, its accent, the words. And then *Abuela*'s face began to waver and blur like a television channel about to go out. And then the world behind *Abuela*'s face began to break apart, too, in massive chunks all around them, the sky, the desert, coming apart like a massive galleon being blown apart by cannonball after cannonball while they stood on ship's deck, splintered wood scattering everywhere, their death seeming imminent.

The old woman's voice cut in, asking "What's your name, *m'ija?* How old are you?"

But Luz couldn't remember anything: not her name, not her age, not where she was, not even why her face hurt.

Luz stood there mute and stiff.

"*Bueno*," said the old woman. She took Luz's hand in hers, then whispered tenderly, "Come with me. I'll take you to the border. I'm sure that's where you're heading."

Hand in hand, the two began to walk slowly, the old woman carrying Luz's muddy, empty pink backpack over her humped shoulder. And after about an hour of walking in silence like this, a truck's headlights washed over them.

Before they knew it, a truck had stopped beside them, and a man's nasal voice called out from the darkness "*Buenos días*, where you headed?"

"Laredo," replied the old woman. "*Y juntas.*"

"*Bien*," he yelled back. "Hop in!"

***

In the back of the pick-up, Luz leaned into the old woman, who embraced her. For the first time in many days, she felt loved and safe, as if it were Abuela with her, protecting her, shielding her from the cold air as they sped towards the border with the United States, that final barrier, that threshold between life and death.

Luz fell asleep, and about ninety minutes later, she woke to dawn cracking the horizon, the sky blushing the mildest shade of pink. The truck slid to a dusty stop in a sandy pullout off the highway beside a wide green river.

"Here we are, ladies," called out that nasal male voice, and Luz and the old woman climbed down, thanking the driver, who promptly resumed his journey, disappearing like a cloud of smoke hit by sudden wind.

"The river is called *el Río Grande*," the old woman was saying, "and this side is *Nuevo Laredo, México*; that side *Laredo, Estados Unidos*. You can wade in it for a bit, but then you'll need to swim, and there's a current. Ok?"

"*Sí*," Luz answered, though she hadn't tried to swim in years, not since Tío Marcos had let her into the pool after hours one summer night at the hotel where he'd lucked into some seasonal work as a groundskeeper in San Salvador. How they giggled in the moonlight hurrying to the pool, trying not to get caught by the security guard. How the water had surprised her with how warm it was after being heated all day by the glorious Salvadoran sun. That night seemed eons ago. A life she could never return to. Her head pounded with pain.

"*Bien*," said the old woman. "Get going, *m'ija*. The later it gets, the sunnier it gets, too, making it easier for *La migra* to see you. Be careful. I'll watch you set off, and then I'm heading into Juárez to see my sister. *Suerte, m'ija*."

The old woman hugged Luz, then crossed her, saying "*Que dios te bendiga*."

Luz took this as a sign to go and so began to shuffle away, down the sandy path to the river's edge.

The noise in her head whirred its high-pitched ring, and her face pulsated with pain, and she felt as if her body were moving without her, separated from her mind, her spirit. In one last act of resistance, her brain told her to stop, but then it flashed Kelvin's face behind her eyelids. She saw his silver-toothed sneer, heard the gunshots, and as they echoed in her head, she plunged into the frigid river.

***

Coughing, twisting, kicking, Luz writhed in the *Rio Grande*. She couldn't see. Couldn't tell where the sky was. Where to try to swim. Her nausea surged. The ringing in her head was so loud that she thought her head would explode with the shrieking. She splashed and fought and spun gagged in the rushing current, but she couldn't break free. *El Río Grande* had her. She was pinned in its grip. She remembered Kelvin's hard hands on her shoulders, pinning her in place. She remembered the stale stench of his breath, the taste of his blood when she'd bitten him. But this time there was no freeing herself. This time she was trapped, hoping to pass out and die just to stop the agony, the ringing, the retching, when from nowhere a pole appeared in front of her.

She grabbed it. From somewhere she could hear distant shouting, muffled words. Blind, exhausted, ready to die in this frigid river, she nevertheless held tight, which was no small feat. It required every ounce of energy in her ninety-pound, famished body. She closed her eyes hard to hold on tighter, and soon she realized she was being pulled through the current towards the far shore.

The distant shouting was getting louder. Soon the tops of her toes scraped the sandy riverbed, and a man who looked like a police officer in a green uniform dropped his end of the pole and rushed to her in the shallows. She noticed his eyes go wide when he reached her, seeing her exposed nose, her last surgical mask having been torn away in the river.

He moved quickly, lifting her from the water and cradling her in his arms as if she weighed little more than a child's doll. As he splashed towards shore, she looked into his face, which looked familiar: caramel skin, black hair, a thin moustache like Tío Edilber's, but she couldn't understand the words coming out of his mouth. She thought it was because he was talking into her deaf ear. And then she fainted.

**

Luz woke in a hospital bed with white sheets, white blankets, and a white pillow beneath her knees. There was an IV in her arm, white lights burning above her, and a beeping machine next to her good ear.

Looking down she noticed she was dressed in a blue hospital gown and two yellow socks, nothing more, making her feel exposed, vulnerable, alone, afraid.

"Am I going into surgery again? Did the green policeman shoot me in the head? Where am I? Where's *Mamá?*"

And, ¡*uf!*, her head. It throbbed, as brutally as ever. And it still burned with that piercing ringing, though her nausea was conspicuously minimal.

"Where am I? What's happening?"

Another green policeman appeared. This one spoke Spanish.

"*¿Cómo te llamas, m'ija?*"

**

This green policeman had told her his name was Fabián, and he had kind, brown eyes like a chocolate Labrador Retriever's, and his frame was bulky, solid with muscles. Feeling safe enough, or at least sheltered in her exhaustion, Luz finally let her guard down, gave in. She began to blurt out everything to Fabián, as if in confessional, intimating the entirety of her migration story to him: how Abuela had needed chicken, how she'd wanted red lipstick, how excited she'd been to meet her tíos' girlfriends, how Kelvin had appeared, how he was a feared mara leader, how he'd always fancied young girls like her, how he'd ruined everything by trying to touch her, how she'd bitten his finger, how his blood tasted holt and salty, how she'd turned to run, how he'd shot two bullets into her head and fled, leaving her for dead, how she'd woken in heaven or a hospital like this one, everything white and clean.

Fabián wrote it all down in a small black notebook, his pen moving furiously as she spoke and spoke until running out of energy, and when she was finally silent, he simply said "You did well, Luz. Now get some rest. You're safe here. We'll take good care of you."

With that she realized just how soft the pillow was beneath her aching head, and she felt how the feathery mattress beneath her made her feel as if she'd sunken in a sunlit cloud. Within seconds she was asleep, her first real, deep sleep in weeks. She even dreamed.

***

Luz didn't understand. What was happening? Was she still asleep? Was this a dream? Why was this man in a suit and tie handcuffing her to her hospital bed?

"What's happening?" she asked, sitting up, her head surging with so much pain she gagged, trying to keep from vomiting.

"Luz Esperanza," the main in the suit said sternly through an interpreter, "you're being detained as a stateless criminal alien. A federal judge has determined your ties to MS-13 to make you a threat to the public and to yourself, too. He has therefore remanded you to our custody, and you'll be placed in a maximum-security detention center, where you'll be housed for the duration of your immigration case, which we hope to resolve within three months, though it could take up to a year, occasionally longer."

***

The next morning Luz was shackled and whisked by van from the hospital to a maximum-security detention center three states away, where a female police officer in a black uniform took custody of her, marched her through a series of locked gates then doors, and finally into a small, windowless room, which was so humid and musty Luz felt like she barely could breathe.

There the officer stripped Luz naked—the first time she'd ever been naked in front of a stranger. Luz tried to cover herself with her trembling hands as the officer methodically looked into Luz's eyes, ears, and every orifice, before pushing a gray sweat suit at the humiliated girl and indicating that she should dress, and quickly.

While getting dressed, Luz couldn't think straight. Her head pounded with the usual pain, and the all-too-familiar buzzing raged between her ears. Through it all she tried softly to ask for a surgical mask. "To cover my nose." But the officer failed to respond, either unable to understand Spanish or choosing to ignore it.

The officer brusquely grabbed Luz's sweatshirt between her shoulder blades and began to walk her out of the exam room and down a long, silent corridor, where, nose exposed, Luz stared at the white ceiling, its fluorescent tubes of lighting, and tried not to cry. "Not now, not here."

At the end of the corridor, the officer pushed Luz to the right, and they passed through another locked door, which opened to a cavernous white hall whose perimeter was lined with perfectly spaced-out individual jail cells. Each had a windowless, blue metal door, and Luz noticed the third door on the left was open. That was exactly where they headed. Arriving at the door, the officer pushed Luz through, and then Luz heard the door close and lock her in.

"What's happening?" Luz asked.

No one answered.

She looked around. The room was little more than a concrete box with a metal toilet and a metal plank for a bed. Sealed in it, she felt a claustrophobic terror rise in her throat like a scream. And then it rang out, surprising Luz, filling the tiny space, a howl so horrible and piercing she could scarcely believe it was coming from her. It was the sound of suffocating in isolation. The sound of being a child utterly alone. The sound of surviving an attempted rape. The sound of *La Bestia* ripping through Mexico. The sound of death beckoning her in the desert. The sound of not being home.

***

Later that afternoon—two hours later? four? six? — she woke to the clatter of her cell door being opened.

A new officer, this time a towering man, waited backlit in the doorframe, his hands on his hips. His massive silhouette seemed to seethe, and she understood not to make him wait.

"Get up," he barked in Spanish with a strange, twangy accent, almost incomprehensible.

Luz obeyed. Like *abuela* always said, Luz was nothing if not a good girl.

She followed the giant figure out into the cavernous hall, through its front door, and then back down the long corridor, but to a new room. Therein a small, bespectacled man in a nice suit and tie was sitting at a table with a tape-recorder on it, waiting for her.

With a wave he indicated that she should sit down in the empty chair across the table from him. He then punched the red button on a voice recorder, laid it on the table between them, and leaned forward.

Luz held her breath. Her face throbbed, and the high-pitched buzz in her head was as loud as it had ever been. The man cleared his throat, smoothed his dark red tie, and looked straight into the hole where she'd once had a beautiful Mayan nose.

"15 December 2016," he said into the recorder. "9:15am. I'm in the Grand Heights Juvenile Detention Center to interview a new detainee, Luz Esperanza Flores Martínez."

"Luz Esperanza," he then said in perfect Spanish. "I'm Special Investigator LeGrange, and I want you to tell me everything you know about your gang, MS-13."

Luz must've looked as baffled as she felt. Her stomach knotted, and she couldn't speak. "Was this some kind of *gringo* joke? Did I not hear him correctly? Had he spoken into my deaf ear? Gang? MS-13? Me?"

"Ok, then," he said, visibly frustrated. "Let's start with something easier. Tell me, Luz Esperanza: why did you come to the United States?"

Buscando a Luz
Wendy Herrera (Translator)

Esa mañana en el taller de poesía Luz me dijo que no podía creer su buena suerte: Abuela le había dado diez dólares para que comprara pollo, también le dijo que podía comprarse un lápiz labial con el cambio. Y cambio habría. Con su burbujeante entusiasmo esa mañana de verano, Luz salió corriendo de su apartamento de una habitación en Soyopango, San Salvador, sabiendo exactamente qué color de lápiz labial quería. Era un tono rojo, rojo carmín, profundo y lustroso como el de un jocote que está siendo besado por el sol, el mismo color que Susana, la chica más popular de la escuela, había debutado la semana pasada, causando furor entre las chicas de su clase de noveno grado en la escuela Panamericana.

"Date prisa, Luz" le había dicho Abuela, hizo pasar a la adolescente por la puerta dándole una cariñosa palmadita en el trasero, esta atesorada nieta, la única de Abuela, y por eso mimaba a la niña, como con el lápiz labial. Se lo merece, Abuela pensó, viendo como Luz se alejaba saltando. *Es tan dulce, tan buena, Gracias, Dios, por esta gran bendición.*

Y con esto Abuela regresó a la cocina para continuar preparando el almuerzo semanal familiar de los domingos en su departamento, donde vivía con Luz y su madre, y donde los otros dos hijos de Abuela, los tíos de Luz llegarían pronto para comer con ellas.

Eran una familia pequeña pero feliz, unida y tierna, una rareza en cualquier parte del mundo, y especialmente en este vecindario plagado de pandillas y drogadictos y policías abusivos que constantemente ahuyentaban a la gente o los envían a la cárcel, destrozando familias.

En contra de tal ruptura, la familia de Luz parecía crecer: justo en esa mañana, Tío Marcos y Tío Edilber llamaron a Abuela para preguntar si podían llevar a sus novias a almorzar, asegurando, un augurio prometedor.

"Claro, m'ijo," ella les había contestado a cada uno de ellos con alegría en su voz. "Siempre hay lugar. Hay lugar para todos".

De ahí la necesidad de más pollo al último minuto, y Abuela sabía que Luz era buena para eso. Ella era inteligente y rápida como un conejo, tanto en casa como en la escuela. Ay, *tesoro mío*, pensó Abuela, sonriendo mientras amasaba la masa para las pupusas.

Mientras tanto, Luz ya estaba afuera, saltando por la calle hacia el mercado Súper Selecto, sus trenzas negras azabache se mecían sobre su espalda como si estos fueran sus sellos de felicidad, estás haciendo volteretas y giros. Ella pensaba en el lápiz labial mientras se tocaba el billete aterciopelado en el bolso, colgado diagonalmente sobre el pecho para mayor seguridad.

Mientras se apresuraba, la luz de aquella mañana era tan brillante que la hizo entrecerrar los ojos, lo que hizo que se diera cuenta, que había olvidado sus gafas de sol en su apuro.

"Rayos", ella pensó. "Un golpe doble". No solo tendría que soportar el duro resplandor de la luz con sus ojos descubiertos, sino que también tenía que caminar en público sin gafas, ya que estas rompían el largo óvalo de su rostro. Este fue un truco de belleza que había aprendido hace dos meses en un artículo en una revista femenina- "Consejos de moda para el verano 2016"- y lo había practicado religiosamente desde entonces, después de haberse preocupado con la típica inseguridad adolescente de que su cara era horrible, monstruosamente enorme y carnosa, su característica más fea.

Mirando hacia abajo para evitar la luz y ocultar su rostro, Luz siguió adelante, sintiéndose cohibida, conspicua, a solo tres cuadras del Súper Selecto.

"¡Tan Cerca! ¡Casi llego!" Y esperaba no ver a nadie que conociera y tener que parar y hacer algún tipo de conversación, cuando todo lo que quería hacer, era perderse en el pasillo de maquillaje. "¿Rojo mágico o rojo místico?", se preguntaba, ya de compras en su cabeza, mientras el suave dobladillo de su falda floreada se movía detrás de ella, en un viento de cola, marcando su velocidad y propósito.

Y así, perdida en sus pensamientos, apresurándose mientras miraba hacia abajo, casi tropezaba con alguien que venía directamente hacia ella en la acera. Kelvin, *Uh oh*.

"Mira, chica, mira para dónde vas", dijo sin rodeos, pero con una sonrisa, mostrando un diente incisivo de plata que brillaba.

"Perdón" Luz murmuró a través de una mueca avergonzada, mirando hacia abajo otra vez.

Intentó esquivar a Kelvin y continuar su viaje, pero él también trato de esquivarla, como si fuese reflejo de su cuerpo. Luego la agarró con fuerza por los hombros y la miró de arriba abajo, mirándola con lascivia.

"Daaamn, niña", le dijo. "Te ves bien. Toda crecida y mierda".

Luz se estremeció. Kelvin dirigía la clica local de MS-13. Todos sabían evitarlo.

Había pasado tres años en la cárcel, donde se rumoreaba que había matado a dos personas, y él siempre estaba afuera robando, golpeando, intimidando y lamiendo sus labios.

Luz quería alejarse rápidamente, pero el agarre en sus hombros era firme.

"¿Qué te pasa, Luz?" preguntó.

La pregunta la hizo sentir como si hubiera un desprendimiento de rocas detrás de sus costillas.

"¿Tienes miedo de mí, niña?", Preguntó, lamiendo su plateado diente incisivo. "¡Bueno, no lo tengas! Te trataré bien".

"Es que tengo prisa", ella respondió rápidamente, tratando de liberarse, de evadirlo. Pero él la sostuvo, y la ardiente luz de aquel día, hacía que su cabeza calva se mirará como si estuviera envuelta en llamas.

Comenzó a girar la cabeza, mirando largo y tendido arriba y abajo de la cuadra. Luz vio el tatuaje de calavera en su cuello estirarse y comprimirse mientras se movía, como si fuera una especie de fantasma compinche, ayudándolo.

Rápidamente como el golpe de una víbora, Kelvin puso una mano en los labios sin pintar de Luz y la arrastró hacia el callejón adyacente abandonado, al no ser por una bolsa de plástico que rodaba en una suave brisa.

Los ojos de Luz se llenaron de miedo. Se bloqueó, apenas podía respirar.

"Sí, te ves bien, niña", murmuraba mientras la arrastraba detrás de un contenedor de basura, una mano todavía amordazaba su boca, la otra recorría su muslo y debajo de su falda, hasta que gritó de dolor.

"Perra, ¿Por qué me muerdes?", rugió, con sus ojos oscuros comprimidos como si fueran viciosas hendiduras, mientras sacudía y agitaba su mano ensangrentada en el aire, furioso, saltando de dolor. "¡Perra, te voy a matar!"

Con su mano sana, sacó una pistola de su cintura, y Luz, finalmente pudo moverse, giró para correr, antes de caer en su lugar, con dos balas en la cabeza.

***

"M'ija, tienes que irte", decía la madre de Luz entre lágrimas. "Te tienes que irte para el norte, a los Estados Unidos. Es la única forma, m'ija. Por favor."

"No puedo, mamá", sollozaba Luz, "No voy a ir. No puedo hacerlo".

Su madre la estrechó en un suave abrazo, y las dos sollozaron y lloraron, paradas, allí justo en el medio de la sala de Abuela.

Mamá lloró y sollozó con la idea de perder a su única hija, su preciosa Luz.

Luz sollozó y lloró a pesar de que su cabeza latía con un dolor incandescente. Sentía como si alguien le estuviera quemando con una espiga de metal en la oreja izquierda, y se la pasaban por la cara hasta llegar a su nariz. Y el dolor en su corazón era aún peor.

Sollozaba y sollozaba, aunque seguía sorda de un oído y un zumbido agudo llenaba su cabeza incesantemente, por no mencionar el mareo, la náusea, los repentinos ataques de vómito.

Ella había estado así durante días, pero los médicos insistieron en que estaba lista para irse a casa. Habían dicho una y otra vez en el hospital, que había tenido suerte. "Has tenido mucha suerte, Luz" Ellos dijeron. "Eres una chica muy afortunada". Y luego se quedaron allí sonriéndole, satisfechos consigo mismos, como si lo hubieran arreglado todo.

Al principio, ella les creyó, a pesar de un dolor constante que a veces aumentaba tan repentinamente que el dolor la segaba temporalmente, como un rayo masivo, la agonía hacia que cayera de rodillas. "Una chica muy afortunada". Seguían insistiendo.

"Una limpieza absoluta", lo llamaron, mostrándole los rayos-X, dónde había entrado la primera bala, detrás de la oreja izquierda y luego saliendo de la fosa nasal izquierda. "El mejor resultado posible teniendo en cuenta la ubicación. En ocasiones, una bala rebota en el cuerpo y causa todo tipo de daños".

A la misma vez, se maravillaron con la segunda bala: cómo milagrosamente había sido menos intrusiva, menos dañina, cómo esta se había alojado entre el cuero cabelludo y el cráneo en la coronilla de la cabeza, detenida en seco, por así decirlo. Antes de poder desgarrar su cerebro.

"Ay, m'ija", su madre la arrullaba, "Ya lo sé. Lo sé, lo sé". Su susurro sonaba decaído, herido, distante.

"Si Kelvin descubre que sobreviviste", intervino Abuela, "volverá para matarte, m'ija. No es una broma, y no hay discusión posible. Usted se tiene que ir. Te vas a ir".

Detrás de la máscara quirúrgica que cubría su nariz desfigurada, Luz sintió que estaba desapareciendo, desmoronándose por dentro. Su cabeza fuertemente vendada temblaba sobre su frágil cuerpo, ella temblaba de miedo. No podía irse. Simplemente esto no era posible. Ni siquiera quería dejar ir el abrazo de su madre, y mucho menos el departamento, el sofá desplegable que compartía con su madre desde su nacimiento, el único hogar que había conocido. Y ahora tenía que dejarlo, ¿salir de Soyopango, salir de El Salvador?

"No puedo", sollozó. "No puedo, Mamá. No puedo hacerlo".

Pero también sabía que tenía que hacerlo, o Kelvin o alguno de sus secuaces la matarían.

***

Toda la familia –Abuela, Mamá, Tío Marcos, Tío Edilber, y Luz— se reunieron melancólicamente en la mesa del comedor esa noche, para reunir el dinero para el viaje a los Estados Unidos.

"¿Cuatrocientos cincuenta y tres dólares?", preguntó Tío Edilber mientras terminaba de contarlo todo. "¿Eso es todo lo que tenemos?" movió la cabeza.

Todos guardaron silencio, sabiendo que esto no era suficiente. Incluso, aunque, ella viajará de gratis a través de México en la Bestia. Luz aún necesitaría al menos mil dólares para sentirse mínimamente cómoda y segura para viajar. Pero esto era todo lo que tenían, y ella tenía que marcharse. Ya había rumores de que Kelvin había oído hablar de su existencia.

Nadie habló. Abuela acarició la espalda de Luz, mientras la niña lloraba silenciosamente a su lado.

"Escucha, Luz", dijo Tío Marcos, fingía una sonrisa mientras hablaba. "Cuando llegues a Gringolandia, ellos te arreglarán bien. Ellos tienen los mejores doctores del mundo. ¡Te harán ver como Shakira, si tu quieres!".

Pero su gentil gesto fracasó, y su voz se disolvió en la pesadez de la habitación, como una pizca de azúcar que se disuelve en el té negro.

"Mañana por la mañana, m'ija" decía Mamá. "Es porque te amo. Es porque te amamos, porque eres más fuerte de lo que tú crees".

***

A la mañana siguiente, a las siete, Luz, con una mochila rosada y una manzana, una banana y una botella de agua subió al autobús en la Terminal de Occidente.

El boleto le había costado 36 dólares, menguando su presupuesto, pero esta pérdida no era tan grande como la que llevaba en su corazón, el cual iba cayendo en espiral, en un pozo aparentemente sin fondo, que sonaba similar al ruido estridente que continuamente llenaba su cabeza desde la cirugía, como si fuera la banda sonora de su vida desde el tiroteo.

Luz subió al autobús y se sentó, ella se sentía como si estuviera fuera de su cuerpo, ella sentía como si se mirará a sí misma. Se sentía hueca, liviana, con un remolino de confusión, de soledad y de miedo. La mezcla recorrió por su cuerpo, haciéndola temblar. Ella sentía como si estuviera atrapada en una ducha helada. Su cabeza latía como siempre, con el dolor palpitante, y muy apenas notó las lagrimas que recorrían por sus mejillas y recorrían la máscara quirúrgica que ocultaba su nariz desfigurada.

Mientras el motor del autobús rugía a la vida, no pudo soportar mirar la ventana, donde estaba su familia, quienes se habían reunido en la acera, al otro lado de la ventana, para despedirse de ella. En lugar de eso, bajó la vista a su regazo y vio caer las gotas de sus lágrimas sobre sus rodillas, como en cámara lenta. Sus manos temblaban, tanto que decidió sentarse sobre ellas, y en esa postura comenzó a alejarse.

Sola en el asiento de su ventana, parecía tan pequeña, tan vulnerable, como un niño pequeño que se está ahogando en el centro de un lago enorme, que es inalcanzable.

Anhelaba estar otra vez en el sofá abultado de Abuela, riéndose de las novelas con ella.

"¿Cómo voy a sobrevivir sin ella? ¿Sin Mamá? ¿Sin mis tíos? ¿Cuándo los volveré a ver?"

El autobús salió de la estación a sacudidas y a borbotones, era la primera parada de los siguientes serpenteantes tres días llenos de paradas que con suerte llevarían a Luz a Tapachula, Chiapas.

***

Estaba completamente oscuro y frio cuando Luz se despertó. "¿Acaso he perdido la vista?", se preguntó, sin ver nada al principio, hasta que el mundo volvió lentamente a ella, la oscuridad se disolvía.

Su máscara quirúrgica estaba pegada a su nariz destrozada, por causa de la sangre seca, le dolía al ajustarla. Le dolía la cabeza, con el dolor habitual, ya estaba habituada al sonido áspero, ese dolor ruido constituían sus únicos dos compañeros en este viaje, las únicas cosas familiares, predecibles, conocidas.

"Dios mío, susurró." No puedo hacer esto. "No soy lo suficientemente fuerte. Dios, llévame de aquí."

Luz no tenía idea de dónde estaba, o qué hora era, o qué haría si Dios la obligara a vivir esta pesadilla antes del amanecer. Ella estaba hambrienta. Ella estaba cansada. Ella estaba asustada y sola y en agonía física.

Luz quería ceder y abandonar este viaje imposible, ser revocada de la tierra hasta el cielo por Dios, el cielo, cielo oscuro de su alrededor, envolviéndola, tragándosela al dulce olvido.

En ese momento, la mano cálida de una anciana guatemalteca se deslizó en la de Luz, entrelazando sus dedos. La anciana, como por arte de magia, levantó a Luz de su asiento y la llevó al pasillo con ella.

Paradas allí, en la silenciosa oscuridad, se miraron a los ojos. Luz vio como radiaba de sus ojos la amabilidad, la anciana vio el dolor de Luz. Era tan obvio como común en los niños que viajaban por esta ruta, especialmente cuando estaba solos, y en los últimos años, la anciana lo había visto en los ojos de miles de jóvenes migrantes: guatemaltecos, hondureños, salvadoreños, nicaragüenses, todos pasando por su estado natal, San Marcos, que ella misma recorría todos los días; vendiendo tamales caseros en una cesta de plástico envuelta en una manta, de parada en parada de autobús, para ganarse el pan de cada día.

"Ven conmigo, m'ija", dijo suavemente, con cuidado de no asustar a la chica con el ruido.

Envuelta en varios suéteres y una bufanda desteñida, la anciana llevó a Luz afuera del autobús en Melacatán, la última parada en Guatemala, desolada en aquella pauta antes del amanecer, excepto por algunos pocos conductores de autobuses fumando cigarrillos y un grupo de pasajeros soñolientos dando vueltas en la estación para mantenerse calientes, en estas horas finales y frías antes del amanecer.

Ella puso un tamal caliente en la mano de Luz, y el repentino calor, se extendió a través de los dedos de Luz, que, rígidos y apretados por el frio, comenzaron a aflojarse, abriéndose en forma de una orquídea que se despliega en el calor húmedo. La calidez viajaba por el brazo de Luz, hasta llegar a su pecho, donde se alojaba como un pequeño amanecer, como una estrella nueva, que, en lo profundo de su cuerpo, reavivaba una pequeña esperanza.

"Si no tienes papeles, mi amor", le susurró la anciana a Luz, acariciando su mano, "entonces es mejor caminar una cuadra hacía arriba, alrededor de ese edificio, ¿Lo ves? Un poco más allá, hay un callejón. Síguelo hasta llegar a un campo, cruza la alcantarilla y allí encontrarás un lecho de río seco. Si puedes cruzarlo en la oscuridad, evitarás que te vean. Incluso podrás ver a otros allí, haciendo lo mismo. No tengas miedo. Solo sigue moviéndote".

Ella le estaba susurrando tan suave que Luz apenas podía escucharla, incluso cuando dirigía su mejor oreja directamente a los labios de la anciana y se inclinaba hacia ella.

"Eres mi ángel, mi vida", creyó haber escuchado a la anciana decir a modo de conclusión.

A la misma vez, Luz sabía lo desorientada que se sentía, que tan enfermizo era ese dolor. Su rostro palpitaba, su cabeza resonaba, y estaba aterrada y aturdida por el miedo. Además, estaba hambrienta, tenía sed y necesitaba orinar. Entonces, ella simplemente asintió y susurró: "Gracias, Señora".

"Está bien", dijo la anciana. "Ten cuidado, Ten cuidado, m'ija. Hay ladrones en todas partes, incluso con insignias y porras. Ve ahora, m'ija. Se rápida e invisible".

Y Luz se fue.

***

Al recordar su viaje de 1,450 millas desde Tapachula a Monterrey encima de La Bestia, el Tren de la Muerte, todo lo que Luz pudo recordar fue la angustia. Durante las 1,450 millas del viaje, ella rebotó en el techo de los vagones de carga, hombro a hombro con otras personas sentadas ahí; la lluvia y el viento y el sol los castigaba, expuestos día y noche. Aunque las noches, a menudo, eran mucho peor debido al frío feroz ya fuera del bosque, o de la jungla, o del desierto. Era la forma en que el sol caía, este caía como un boleto de lotería fallido, otra oportunidad pérdida para ver el nuevo mundo. Otro día de suciedad, de hambre, de exposición, volviendo a la desolación oscura de una noche, para estremecerse con los soñadores que estaban exhaustos, que lentamente se deshidrataban, perdiendo la esperanza y la energía.

Sí, las noches definitivamente habían sido las peores: hora tras hora, se sentía como si se bañara en agua helada bajo un fuerte ventilador que nunca dejaba de soplar. Se sentía como si témpanos de hielo en forma de espadas se empujaran a través de su pecho y garganta, una y otra vez. Y algunas veces dormía, y a menudo se despertaba al ser sobada en la oscuridad, por los hombres sibilantes: manoseaban sus pechos, muslos y nalgas; la pellizcaban y la arañaban, la pellizcaban y la agarraban. En una ocasión, se había despertado con labios excitados y pegajosos que se movían de arriba a abajo por su cuello como babosas. Cada vez que esto sucedía, ella se ponía tiesa del terror, incapaz de gritar, y mucho menos de huir. Luz muda como una estatua, Luz castigada por este repetido abuso, mientras se movían hacía el norte.

Peor aún, cada vez que esto sucedía, veía el rostro de Kelvin esquematizado en cada uno de sus abusadores. Kelvin, gruñendo con ese diente de plata. La mano de Kelvin debajo de su falda. El estallido de dos disparos rápidos, el despertar del dolor en el hospital, el dolor punzante que cada vez sentía cuando tenía que quitarse la máscara quirúrgica de la cara, donde la sangre seca cubría su nariz destrozada.

Además, había hambre en La Bestia. El hambre, como nunca la había conocido. Un agujero en su vientre, en el que sentía como si todo su ser fuera constantemente arrastrado hacía dentro, el hambre por olvidar, el tornado sin fin, y se reducía su voluntad por vivir.

Y ella no podía hacer nada. En su primer día, en lo alto del tren, compró dos bolsas de papas fritas, lo que la dejó sedienta. Una hora más tarde, vio a un niño aparecer sobre su automóvil, vendiendo sodas y agua, compró una Fanta naranja en bolsa. Pero en lugar de la soda, él sacó un machete y le exigió su bolso, y rápidamente huyó. Otros sabían del niño, un marero del área, pero nadie le había advertido a Luz.

Hacia el final del viaje, cada vez que el tren se detenía, se bajaba y buscaba basura para comer, y si no podía encontrar ninguna, se tiraba y mascaba hierba como una cabra fuera de control, sintiendo vergüenza profunda, y se preguntaba en voz alta, si ella todavía era un ser humano.

***

La última vez que Luz saltó de La Bestia, estaba finalmente a las afueras de Monterrey, Nuevo León, dejándole unas 200 millas para llegar a Laredo, Texas, el famoso Estados Unidos, la Tierra de la Libertad.

Pero Luz no estaba segura de poder conseguirlo. Ella estaba agotada, sucia, sin un centavo en la bolsa, y desesperadamente sola. Su cabeza aún latía con el dolor que parecía una bomba, una bomba explotando una y otra vez de su nariz. Y todavía estaba sorda de un oído, cambiando su relación con el mundo exterior, y dentro de su cabeza, el zumbido penetrante y habitual borraba cualquier intento de organizar sus ideas, o de calmar sus nervios.

Ella comenzó a rascarse los antebrazos, debajo de su ropa sucia, que le había resacado la piel y la había producido picazón. Su cuero cabelludo también picaba, allí debajo de su pelo grueso y enmarañado con grasa, suciedad y sudor seco, aunque no se atrevía a rascarse por temor a arrancarse las costras de las heridas de las balas, y comenzar a sangrar nuevamente; esta vez sin nada que pararlo, nada para detenerlo.

Y así, ella se alejó del autobús, sintiéndose horrible, monstruosa, abandonada por la humanidad, por Dios, por Jesús, y por la Virgen de Guadalupe. Había abandonado el plan que Tío Marcos había trazado para ella en este punto de la travesía, tenía que haber hecho un autostop por la carretera 85 hasta la frontera, tal vez, incluso cruzar en carro, si tenía suerte, con una familia chicana con documentos, que viajarán de regreso a los Estados Unidos, mezclándose con ellos, para escabullirse a través de un punto de control, con una sonrisa de inocencia tímida.

Pero no. Ese era un plan para una Luz diferente, la de una época diferente, que apenas podía recordar. Así que, en lugar de dirigirse a la carretera, Luz se desvió de su curso, y se dirigió al desierto más cercano, desolado, excepto por la creosota, los cactus y un zopilote solitario que daba vueltas a la distancia.

Mientras tanto, sus compañeros de viaje del autobús partieron hacia el norte en grupos para buscar su destino. Luz los escuchó irse, sabía la dirección correcta, pero no podía reunir las fuerzas para seguirlos, para seguir creyendo.

Después de haber recorrido algunos cien metros, se dejó caer en la arena, detrás de un antiguo saguaro, su coraje había sido consumido por tantos días de hambre, de abuso y por el castigo de la soledad.

Atormentada por el dolor y la angustia, agotada, se metió un puñado de arena en la boca y masticó, esperando que esto la ayudará a disolverse en el desierto, que se deslizara en una muerte pacífica en ese mismo lugar, que transportaran su espíritu a algún lugar, donde su cabeza no le doliera, en donde no pudiera ser manoseada, robada o golpeada.

Masticaba lentamente, se abrochó la cremallera de su sudadera con capucha, hasta que dejo un pequeño agujero, luego comenzó a rezar para ser sepultada. Mientras esperaba, se concentró en el dolor palpitante que emanaba de las heridas de las balas en su cabeza y de su nariz destrozada. Comenzó a llorar, una pena profunda y estremecedora, que la sorprendió con la violencia de sus espasmos, de la misma manera de un trueno repentino, que en ocasiones sacude al cielo y luego viene el aguacero explosivo y violento.

***

Nadie sabe cuánto tiempo paso Luz allí acurrucada, sollozando sola en el desierto, de repente apareció una anciana. Esta vez fue Abuela.

"¡Abuela!" Luz gritó, recobrando su juicio.

Ella se levantó del suelo, con una gran sonrisa en su rostro, detrás de su máscara quirúrgica hecha jirones, veteada de sangre seca.

Las dos compartieron un profundo y cálido abrazo, Luz enterró su rosto en el cuello de Abuela y dijo: "Abuela, ¡qué bueno verte! ¡Gracias por venir!"

Entonces la anciana se alejó.

"M'ija", dijo en voz baja. "No soy tu abuela. Mi nombre es Alicia Benítez Rodríguez. Soy mexicana, de esta área".

Luz estaba confundida. Había escuchado las palabras, incluso había notado el extraño acento mexicano con el que hablaba Abuela, pero estaba segura de que su abuela estaba allí, era la misma cara de Abuela, ella reconocería esos ojos brillantes en cualquier lugar, y sus mejillas sonrojadas.

"¿Estás bien, m'ija?" preguntó la anciana, con un chal sobre la cabeza, haciéndola parecer una especie de Santa Abuela en medio del desierto.

Luz no dijo nada, solo se quedó mirando ese rostro familiar. Estaba todavía confundida por la extraña voz, su acento, sus palabras. Entonces la cara de Abuela comenzó a oscilarse y a difuminarse como una canal de televisión a punto de apagarse. Luego, el mundo detrás de la cara de Abuela comenzó a hacerse borroso, en trozos enormes a su alrededor, el cielo y el desierto, deshaciéndose como una embarcación siendo destrozada por una bala de cañón, una tras otra, mientras estaban en la cubierta de la embarcación, astillas de madera en todas partes, y su muerte parecía que era inminente.

La voz de la anciana, la trajo de regresó a la realidad, "¿Cuál es tu nombre, m'ija? ¿Cuántos años tienes?"

Pero Luz no podía recordar nada: ni su nombre, ni su edad, ni dónde estaba, ni siquiera sabía por qué le dolía la cara.

Luz se quedó allí muda y tiesa.

"Bueno", dijo la anciana. Ella tomó la mano de Luz y le susurró con ternura: "Ven conmigo. Te llevaré a la frontera. Estoy segura de que es hacia donde te diriges".

Tomadas de la mano, las dos comenzaron a caminar lentamente, mientras la anciana cargaba la mochila vacía y fangosa de Luz sobre su hombro jorobado. Después de una hora de caminar en silencio de esta manera, los faros de un camión las iluminó.

Antes de darse cuenta, el camión se detuvo junto a ellas, y la voz nasal de un hombre les gritó desde la oscuridad: "Buenos días, ¿A dónde se dirigen?"

"Laredo", respondió la anciana. "Y juntas".

"Bien", les gritó, "¡Súbanse!"

***

En la parte posterior de la camioneta, Luz se inclinó hacía la anciana, que la abrazó. Por primera vez en muchos días, se sintió amada, segura, como si fuera Abuela la que estaba con ella, protegiéndola, sí, protegiéndola del aire frío, mientras se apresuraban hacia la frontera de los Estados Unidos, esa barrera final, ese portal que está entre la vida y la muerte.

Luz se durmió, y unos noventa minutos más tarde, se despertó, con el amanecer rompiendo el horizonte, el cielo ruborizado, con el tono rosado, el más leve que puede haber. El camión se detuvo en aquella explanada arenosa, creando una nube de polvo, junto al ancho río verde.

"Aquí estamos, señoras", les gritó la misma voz nasal masculina, Luz y la anciana bajaron, dándole las gracias al conductor, quien rápidamente reanudó su viaje, desapareciendo como una nube de humo que es golpeada repentinamente por el viento.

"El río se llama El Río Grande", le decía la anciana, "y este lado es Nuevo Laredo, México; aquel lado es Laredo, Estados Unidos. Puedes vadear un poco, pero después, necesitaras nadar y también hay una corriente. ¿De acuerdo?"

"Sí", respondió Luz, aunque no había nadado en años, no desde que Tío Marcos la había dejado entrar a la piscina en la noche, horas después de haber pasado trabajando como jardinero de temporada, donde por suerte había conseguido trabajo aquel verano en el hotel en San Salvador. Cómo se reían a la luz de la luna, corriendo hacia la piscina, tratando de no ser atrapados por el guardia de seguridad. Cómo el agua la había sorprendido con lo cálida que estaba, después de haber sido calentada todo el día por glorioso sol salvadoreño. Aquella noche, parecía que había sucedido hace miles de años. Una vida a la que nunca podría volver. Su cabeza latía de dolor.

"Bien", dijo la anciana. "Ponte en marcha, m'ija. Cuanto más te tardes, más claro se va a poner, haciendo que La Migra te vea con más facilidad. Ten cuidado. Desde aquí te veré partir, y luego me voy a dirigir a Juárez para ver a mi hermana. Suerte, m'ija".

La anciana abrazó a Luz, luego la cruzó, diciéndole a la misma vez, "Que Dios te bendiga".

Luz tomó esto como una señal para irse, y así, comenzó a alejarse, arrastrando los pies por el sendero de arena, hasta la orilla del río.

El ruido en su cabeza zumbó vibrantemente, a la misma vez, su rostro palpitaba de dolor, ella sentía como si su cuerpo se moviera sin ella, como si su
mente estuviera separada de su espíritu. En el último acto de sobrevivencia, su
cerebro le dijo que se detuviera, pero en ese momento, vio la cara de Kelvin
detrás de sus párpados. Vio su diente plateado, escuchó los disparos, y mientras
su cabeza retumbaba, se zambulló en el río helado.

***

Tosiendo y pateando, se retorcía de dolor en El Río Grande. No podía orien-
tarse, no sabía dónde estaba el cielo. Cuando ella trató de nadar, su náusea
aumentó. El zumbido de la cabeza se hacía cada vez más fuerte hasta que pensó
que su cabeza iba a explotar. Ella chapoteó, luchó, y se giró para liberarse de
la corriente, pero no lo logró. El Río Grande la había atrapado, la tenía aga-
rrada firmemente. En ese momento, recordó las duras manos de Kelvin sobre
sus hombros, inmovilizándola. Recordó el hedor rancio de su aliento, el sabor
de su sangre cuando lo mordió. Pero en esta ocasión, estaba atrapada, ella
esperaba desmayarse o morir para poder detener esta agonía, el zumbido, las
náuseas, cuando de la nada apareció un poste enfrente de ella.

Lo agarró. De algún lugar, se escuchaban gritos, a la distancia, palabras
amortiguadas. Ciega, agotada, lista para morir en aquel río gélido; sin embargo,
se mantuvo firme, lo que no fue poca cosa. Esto requería cada onza de energía
en su cuerpo hambriento de noventa libras. Cerró los ojos con fuerza, para
aferrarse, pronto se dio cuenta que estaba siendo arrastrada por la corriente
hacia lo orilla.

Aquellos gritos distantes, cada vez se hacían más fuertes. Pronto, la parte
superior de los dedos de sus pies toco el lecho arenoso del río, y un hombre con
uniforme verde que parecía ser un oficial de policía, dejó caer el extremo del
poste y corrió hacia ella en las aguas poco profundas. Ella notó como sus ojos
se habrían en par en par, cuando este alcanzó a ver su nariz expuesta, porque
su última máscara quirúrgica había sido arrancada por el río.

Él se movió rápidamente, levantándola del agua y acunándola en sus brazos, como si ella pesara poco más que una muñeca. Mientras chapoteaban
hacia la orilla, ella lo miró a la cara, la que parecía familiar: piel de color cara-
melo, pelo negro, un fino bigote como el de Tío Edilber, pero ella no podía
entender las palabras que salían de su boca. Ella pensó que no las entendía,
porque él le estaba hablando en su oído sordo. Y luego se desmayó.

***

Luz despertó en una cama de hospital con sábanas blancas, mantas y una almohada blanca debajo de sus rodillas. Había una vía intravenosa en su brazo, luces blancas flameando sobre ella y una máquina haciendo ruido junto a su oído bueno.

Mirando hacia abajo, notó que estaba vestida con una bata azul de hospital y un par de calcetines amarillos, eso era lo único que llevaba puesto, lo que la hacía sentirse expuesta, vulnerable, sola, y con miedo.

"¿Me van a operar de nuevo? ¿El policía de verde me dispararía en la cabeza? ¿Dónde estoy? ¿Dónde está Mamá?"

Y, ¡uf!, su cabeza. Palpitaba brutalmente, como siempre. Y todavía le ardía, y ese sonido penetrante, aunque la náusea era menor.

¿Dónde estoy? ¿Qué está pasando?

Apareció otro policía de verde. Este hablaba español.

"¿Cómo te llamas, m'ija?"

***

Este policía de verde le había dicho que su nombre era Fabián; tenía unos ojos muy bonitos, marrones, como los de un Labrador Retriever, su cuerpo era voluminoso, sólido con músculos. Sintiéndose los suficientemente segura, o al menos, refugiada, en su agotamiento, Luz finalmente bajó la guardia, y cedió. Comenzó a contarle todo a Fabián, como si estuviera en un confesionario, contándole toda su historia migratoria: cómo Abuela necesitaba pollo, cómo había querido aquel lápiz labial de color rojo, qué tan emocionada había estado al conocer a las novias de sus tíos, cómo había aparecido Kelvin, cómo este era un temido líder de la mara, cómo siempre a este le habían gustado las chicas jóvenes como ella, cómo él arruino todo al tratar de tocarla, cómo ella había mordido su dedo, cómo su sangre sabía a viejo y salado, cómo se había dado la vuelta para correr, cómo le había disparado dos balas en la cabeza y huyó, dejándola por muerta, cómo ella se había despertado en el cielo o en un hospital parecido a este, todo blanco y limpio.

Fabián escribió todo en un pequeño cuaderno negro, su pluma se movía furiosamente, mientras ella hablaba y hablaba hasta quedarse sin energía, y cuando finalmente se quedó en silencio, él simplemente dijo "lo hiciste bien, Luz. Ahora descansa un poco. Estás a salvo aquí. Te cuidaremos bien".

Con esto, ella se dio cuenta lo suave que era la almohada debajo de su dolorida cabeza, ella se sintió como si debajo de ella estuviera un colchón de plumas, como si estuviera hundida en una nube iluminada por el sol. En cuestión de segundo estaba dormida, su primer descanso real y profundo que no había tenido en semanas. Ella incluso soñó.

***

Luz no entendía. ":¿Qué estaba pasando? ¿Estaba todavía dormida? ¿Sería esto un sueño? ¿Por qué este hombre con traje y corbata la estaba esposando a su cama de hospital?"

"¿Qué está pasando?", ella preguntó, sentándose, el dolor de la cabeza era tan inmenso que la hacía atragantarse, y trataba de no vomitar.

"Luz Esperanza", dijo el hombre con traje, duramente con la ayuda de un intérprete, "estás detenida como una apátrida delincuente extranjera. Un juez federal ha determinado tus vínculos con MS-13, por este motivo, la han hecho una amenaza para el público y hacía usted misma. Por lo tanto, la han dejado bajo custodia y será enviada a un centro de detención de máxima seguridad, donde usted permanecerá alojada mientras dure su caso de inmigración, que esperamos resolver dentro de los próximos tres meses, aunque podría tomarnos hasta un año, y en muchas ocasiones toma más tiempo".

***

La mañana siguiente, Luz fue esposada y traslada en camioneta desde el hospital a un centro de detención de máxima seguridad, el cual estaba lejos, a tres estados de distancia, donde un agente de policía con uniforme negro la custodió, la condujo a través de una serie de puertas, que se cerraban tras de ella, y finalmente a una pequeña habitación sin ventanas, que era tan húmeda, tan húmeda que Luz sentía que apenas podía respirar.

Allí, el oficial desnudó a Luz - esta era la primera vez que ella había estado desnuda enfrente de un extraño.

Luz trató de cubrirse con sus manos temblorosas, mientras que el oficial la miraba metódicamente, los ojos, las orejas, y cada orificio de Luz, antes de lanzarle un traje gris a la chica humillada e indicarle que se vistiera, y rápido.

Mientras ella se vestía, Luz no podía pensar con claridad. Su cabeza palpitaba con aquel dolor familiar, y aquel zumbido demasiado familiar que radiaba entre sus oídos. A pesar de todo, trató tranquilamente de pedir una máscara quirúrgica. "Para taparme la nariz". Pero el oficial no respondió, ya sea a causa de ser incapaz de entender español o porque la ignoraba.

El oficial agarró bruscamente la sudadera de Luz de entre sus omóplatos, y comenzó a salir de la sala de revisión hacia un pasillo largo y silencioso, donde, con la nariz expuesta, Luz contempló el techo blanco, sus tubos fluorescentes de iluminación, y trató de no llorar. "Ahora no, no aquí."

Al final del pasillo, el oficial empujó a Luz hacia la derecha, pasando por otra puerta que estaba cerrada con llave, esta los llevaba a una sala blanca y extensa, cuyo alrededor estaba rodeada de celdas individuales, perfectamente alineadas. Cada una tenía una puerta de metal azul, sin ventanas, Luz notó que la tercera puerta a la izquierda estaba abierta. Exactamente a esa fue donde se dirigieron. Al llegar a la puerta, el oficial la empujó, y luego oyó que se cerraba la puerta y la encerraban

"¿Qué está pasando?", Luz preguntó.

Nadie le respondió.

Ella miró a su alrededor. La habitación era poco más que una caja con un inodoro de metal y una tabla de metal para su cama. Encerrada allí, sintió que un claustrofóbico terror le subía por su garganta como un grito. Y luego retumbó, sorprendiendo a Luz y llenando el pequeño espacio, un aullido tan horrible y penetrante que apenas pudo creer que venía de ella. Era el sonido de sofocación en el aislamiento. El sonido de un niño completamente solo. El sonido de haber sobrevivido el intento de una violación. El sonido de La Bestia desgarrando a México. El sonido de la muerte haciéndole señales en el desierto. El sonido de no estar en casa.

***

En esa misma tarde, tal vez - ¿Dos horas después? ¿Cuatro? ¿Seis? - se despertó por el ruido de la puerta de su celda, que se abría.

Un nuevo oficial, esta vez un hombre imponente, esperó recostado en el marco de la puerta, con las manos en las caderas. Con su enorme silueta echaba humos, y ella comprendió que no lo tenía que hacer esperar.

"Levántate" grito en español, con un acento raro, agazapado, casi incomprensible.

Luz obedeció. Como siempre le había enseñado Abuela, Luz no era sino una buena chica.

Ella siguió a la figura gigante hacia el pasillo cavernoso, a través de la puerta principal, y luego retrocedió por el largo pasillo, pero esta vez a una nueva habitación. Allí, había un hombre pequeño y con gafas, vestido con un bonito traje y una corbata, estaba sentando en una mesa con una grabadora, esperándola.

Con una señal, le indicó que debía sentarse en la silla vacía, al otro lado de la mesa. Luego presionó el botón rojo de una grabadora de voz, la puso sobre la mesa y se inclinó hacia delante.

Luz contuvo el aliento. Su rostro palpitaba, y el zumbido agudo en su cabeza se hacía más fuerte, como lo había sido nunca. El hombre se aclaró la garganta, soltó un poco su corbata roja oscura, y miró directamente al agujero donde una vez había tenido una hermosa nariz maya.

"15 de diciembre del 2016", dijo en la grabadora. "9:15 de la mañana. Estoy en el centro de Detención Juvenil de Grand Heights para entrevistar a una nueva detenida, Luz Esperanza Flores Martínez".

"Luz Esperanza", dijo luego en perfecto español. "Soy el investigador especial LeGrange, y quiero que me cuentes todo lo que sabes sobre tu pandilla, MS-13".

Luz debió parecer tan desconcertada como lo estaba por dentro. Su estómago se anudó y ella no podía hablar. "¿Era esto una especie de chiste gringo? ¿O no lo había escuchado correctamente? ¿O me había hablado en mi oído sordo? ¿Pandilla MS-13? ¿Yo?"

"Está bien, entonces", dijo, visiblemente frustrado. "Comencemos con algo más fácil. Dime, Luz Esperanza: ¿Por qué viniste a los Estados Unidos?"

· 2 ·

PALOMA VILLEGAS

Villegas' poem tells her brother's and her own crossing of the border two decades ago. An accompanying image by Paloma Villegas, illustrates this crossing.

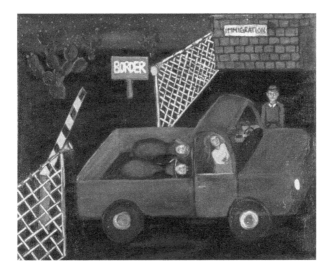

Los Niños Florero, by Paloma E. Villegas (Courtesy of Paloma E. Villegas)

Los niños florero: Cruzaron como floreros

Cuando el oficial de inmigración le preguntó
al conductor si tenía algo
que declarar en su
entrada al país,
el conductor respondió:
"Sí, traigo unos floreros
en la parte trasera de la troca
que voy a usar
para decorar mi casa."
Un niño florero y
Una niña florero

A los niños florero
les dijeron que se durmieran,
que no hicieran ruido
aunque también, la esposa del conductor
había pedido prestado dos actas de nacimiento
de unos niños de la edad de los niños florero.

La niña florero juro no dormirse mientras cruzaban,
hacerse la dormida solamente
para no perderse los acontecimientos.
Pero el sueño le ganó.

Mientras tanto
la mamá
cruzó por la línea,
separada de ellos.
Angustiada pensaba:
¿Qué pasaría si no la dejaban entrar y a sus hijos sí?
¿Qué pasaría si ella entraba y ellos no?

Aunque cruzaron la frontera,
ella, (la frontera), los persiguió,
necia, incrustándose en los floreros.

Los niños crecieron adentro
de esos floreros fronterizos
luchando por salirse
mientras se estrellaban
a todo momento.

Los niños florero.[1] They Crossed the Border Inside *floreros*

When the immigration officer asked
the driver if he had anything
to declare
upon his entry to the country
the driver responded,
"Yes, I have some *floreros*
in the back of the truck
that I will use
to decorate my house."
A boy *florero* and
a girl *florero*.

The *florero* children
were told to sleep,
to not make a sound
although the driver's wife
had borrowed
birth certificates
of two children with the same age
as the *florero* children.

The girl *florero* swore
not to sleep while they crossed,
to only pretend to sleep
so she would not miss what was about to happen.
But sleep won her over.

While this was happening,
their mother crossed
through the line
separated from them,
and worriedly thought:
What would happen if she couldn't cross but her children did?
What if she was able to enter and they weren't?

Although they did cross the border,
it, the border, followed them
stubborn, encrusting herself in the *floreros*.

The children grew up inside
those border *floreros*
fighting to exit
while they crashed against it
at all times

Note

1. A vase or planter.

· 3 ·

CASSANDRA BAILEY

With her story, "Growing Up Too Fast," Bailey advocates for minors with legitimate claims of persecution who qualify for relief through asylum law, but often do not have guidance, such as legal representation, in immigration courts. The result is that many children are forced to hide in the shadows out of fear, or face the system alone, often losing. The story of Ximena's painful trekking restates the theme of sexual violence that very often pushes young women, like the protagonist, out of their countries.

Growing Up Too Fast

When interviewing children, Bailey found certain recurrent patterns. For example, children started talking about fond family memories. For Ximena, growing up in a small *pueblo* in El Salvador was simple. She was the second eldest of seven children and often helped her *mamá* with household responsibilities, including taking care of her younger siblings, cooking, and cleaning. Her older brother, Edgar, started working in the mountains with their *papá* when he turned 12. Dad and son would often be gone for weeks or months working. Even though she did not see *papá* or Edgar for long periods of time, when they came back it was as if they had never left. They spent their nights together eating family dinners, telling stories, playing *arranca cebolla*,[1] and *tripa chuca*.[2] Their *papá* would always bring back presents: stones of all shapes and sizes, one for each child. Ximena would take each stone and polish it down by the stream near their home. She made necklaces out of the stones using wires and twine she found while helping *mamá* on the farm. Then, when her sister was old enough to take care of the four younger children, Ximena was allowed to travel with her *mamá* to the market. She sold her jewelry alongside the *maíz*, eggs, and sugar they raised on the farm. She loved spending time with *mamá*, but the real treat was getting to watch *televisión* in Sra. Rodríguez's air-conditioned shop.

Bailey also found that poverty often emerged in interviews of adolescent girls and in particular they expressed their wish for belonging in a make-believe television world where money abounds and is wasted. Ximena's home did not have electricity, and Sra. Rodriguez's shop was where she was able to watch *tele*. Her favorite show was about four *amigos* that went to the same school. She had never been to school, but she dreamed of attending class one day, wearing makeup, talking to boys, and wearing *gringa* clothes. They had the prettiest hair and perfect makeup, and all the boys liked them. One day, Ximena melted her little sister's crayon and mixed it with oil to make lipstick, so she could be pretty like the *gringas* on the *tele*. Her mom smelled the melted crayon and gave her *una nalgada* for ruining the only pink crayon they had. However, Ximena kept the glossy creation in a tin under her pillow and planned to debut it at her *quinceañera*, which was only a few weeks away.

Mamá had made her a pink dress, and they planned to attend mass with all the *familia*. They made *pupusas* and cake, and invitations were sent to the extended family. All Ximena wanted for her *quinceañera* was a new pair of shoes. She had only been to one *quinceañera* before, and that was her cousin Isela's. She remembered her cousin wore a tiara and looked exactly like a princess. Ximena's *tía* said she would do her hair just like she did Isela's and would lend Ximena her shoes for the ceremony.

Unfortunately, another common denominator in Bailey's research is the memories of the day children were assaulted. The day of the celebration, Ximena's father took her to the salon where her *tía* worked. It was a cool day. When they arrived at the salon, *tía* explained she had to finish up with a client. Ximena sat outside and *Tía* told her not to wander far. Bored, she strolled about near the salon. She was whistled at by a group of boys, felt afraid, and returned to the salon for her *tía* to do her hair. Once she was done, Ximena made her way to a nearby bar where her father was waiting for her. On her way, she saw the same group of boys who whistled at her earlier, and they called her over. She put her head down and continued walking toward the bar.

After that, Ximena only remembered waking up in a dark room with her hands tied together behind her back and her head throbbing. She heard muffled male voices and began to crawl toward the door. Men came barreling through the door. Ximena saw a young man who had tattoos covering his face and neck. The nails on his hand were sharp and pointy and looked like horns. He was skinny and wore a white tank top. He had a gun in his waistband.

"Write down your parent's phone number!" he yelled pointing a gun to Ximena's head.

She said that they did not own a phone, but he laughed. He hit her in the temple with the gun. Ximena felt her head getting hot and began to pray to *Dios*.

"I live near the mountains on a farm," she uttered between sobs.

"*Puta madre* she's poor," he called to another young man.

Ximena lay trembling before she heard a new voice.

"Tell your mom you're alive," he demanded and held a phone up to Ximena's ear.

"I love you," was all she had time to say.

"You have 24 hours to get the money, otherwise she's dead." And they walked out.

Mamá and *papá* sold all they owned, including the new pair of shoes they had bought Ximena as a surprise for her *quince*. They borrowed from family members, but their response was not quick enough.

Around the same time the next day, four men entered the room, letting in a piercing ray of light. They took turns desecrating her body, violating her, pouring beer on her, and beating her. Ximena began to pray and thought about her family trying to block out all fear.

"We've got the money!" one of them shouted, and shortly after, they put a bag over Ximena's head but they didn't bother covering her naked body. She was carried to an *auto* and transported back to town. The *auto* barely slowed down enough for them to push her out. Her arms were still tied, and her head still covered. Ximena laid there still on the pavement. She could not tell how much time passed before she heard a woman scream.

"*Ayúdeme, por favor*," Ximena yelled. The woman clothed her, gave her food, and called the *policía*. The *policía* arrived within minutes and asked her many questions. Her mind was blank. She had trouble remembering anything.

The police drove her back home. She spent the entire car ride attempting to remember something, anything. As she got out of the car her *familia* came running toward her. Then, Ximena remembered the man with the face and neck tattoos. She described the man's tattoos to the *policía*. They seemed to know who he was, and she felt a wave of relief.

The next couple of months were a blur for her. Ximena's family were at the mercy of a police force that was powerless next to gangs and cartels. The police found the young, tattooed man, but she wished they hadn't. He was a high-ranking member of *La Mara Salvatrucha*, more commonly known as the MS-13. The young man was sentenced to 1 month of jail time. The MS-13 did not know where Ximena lived, but they would have figured it out soon. The day after his sentencing, her *tía* was found dead and the *policía* ruled it an accident. El Salvador was no longer safe for Ximena. She had to leave.

Her family didn't have the financial means to pay for a *coyote*, so they borrowed money again. Ximena begged *papá* to let her try to make the journey without guidance, but she left in the middle of the night with the *coyote* and her favorite stone necklace. Her life was now in the hands of some stranger named Miguel, and she was off to the "Land of Opportunity."

Ximena's migration story involved many risks such as being recognized by MS-13 affiliates, being at the mercy of an unknown guide, and surviving the exhaustion, hunger, and thirst of the journey. She joined a group of seven lead by Miguel. They took a bus all the way to a small *pueblo* in Mexico. They were stopped and searched there by the *policía*, who had them each pay a fee before they could continue on their journey. Miguel advised them to remain calm during these types of searches, but Ximena could feel her knees knocking together and her face sweating. They had been traveling for a couple of days and had been rationing meals in small portions of bread and water. Ximena felt an insatiable hunger and thirst, but knew she had to save some bread for harsher conditions.

They traveled for many days and nights through the desert. They were moving slowly but safely. They saw the bodies of several individuals who tried to conquer the journey too quickly or encountered *Los Zetas*.[3] The stench was unbearable, and Ximena found herself gagging at the smell of rotting carcass in the sun. She worried for another traveler, Marta, and her baby. Marta became very sick and malnourished, faster than the rest of them. Ximena shared her bread with her. Now Ximena was running low on food and had much of the journey to go.

After many days and nights in the desert, the bread was long gone, and water was sparse. Ximena was fading in and out of delirium. By the time they arrived at the *río*, it was nighttime. The air was humid, and the water seemed calm. Ximena knew a new life awaited her on the other side of the river, but she was not totally ready to give up her old one.

They piled onto rafts and were told to sit quietly while the men paddled. They floated slowly across the river, neither wanting to disturb the natural flow of water nor create too much noise. The entry point chosen by the *coyote* was covered by brushwood. He helped each person up onto the land. Marta went first as Ximena held baby Kevin. She carefully grabbed Kevin from Ximena's hands and pulled him close to her. Ximena began to make her ascent but the bush she was using as an anchor came loose from the ground. Her foot slipped, and she was soon fully submerged in water. Miguel quickly grabbed onto her leg and put his index finger vertically over his lips. In silence, they were all officially in the United States and each had their own, separate journey to complete.

The *coyote*'s job was done, and Ximena was now tasked with finding her *mamá*'s cousin. Miguel gave her quarters to use at the nearest pay phone. Using caution, she continued to wander north. She stayed hidden as often as possible and refused to rest until she reached a pay phone. She had no food, no water, and hadn't had a good night of sleep in nearly 2 months. She was filthy and wearing dirty clothing, but her fall into the river had taken away most of her stench. She asked for help finding the nearest pay phone. She encountered a young woman pushing her baby in a stroller down the sidewalk, the woman asked Ximena if she could help. She laughed and said, "pay phone?" and pulled a *celular* out of her pocket, ushering Ximena to use it. She dialed the numbers into the phone and waited for *mamá*'s cousin to answer.

"*Bueno?*"

"Is this Sra. Álvarez?" The other person fell quiet. "Hello? It's me, Mariana's daughter." It was as if she was speaking to a ghost.

"Are you safe? Where are you?" she asked.

Sra. Álvarez gave Ximena the address of a friend nearby, Sra. Huerta. This was a place to stay until Sra. Álvarez's son could come pick her up the next day. Walking toward the address, Ximena took in the scenery; there were many churches and a marquee board read August 28, 2012. She had not realized that her journey took 2 months; it felt like an eternity.

"I'm looking for Sra. Huerta. Sra. Álvarez sent me," Ximena said nervously at the doorstep. A man invited her inside and called for Sra. Huerta, his wife. An older woman of small stature came walking out of the kitchen.

"Just in time! I have prepared *menudo!*" Ximena looked to the man who gave her the go ahead to follow his wife into the kitchen. Ximena was overcome with joy, and she started to become teary-eyed. Sra. Huerta looked at her husband and then turned to her and said, "You are safe here; *buen provecho.*"

Ximena's voice was regaining strength as she told this hopeful part of her story.

Sra. Huerta had given her an outfit and pair of shoes. They spent that morning talking about plans for school, making friends, and working to help pay off the loan her parents took out for her. Alberto arrived in the late afternoon. He was well spoken, well dressed, and well-mannered. He had the nicest car Ximena had ever seen. She was so awestruck by the *auto* that she almost forgot to thank Sra. Huerta and her husband for their hospitality. She climbed into the front seat and explored all the buttons. Alberto could tell Ximena was mesmerized by the unfamiliar gadgets and laughed.

"Pretty cool, eh? I just got it with money I saved up from work," Ximena wanted to work where he worked.

It was a long drive, and Ximena eventually fell asleep. He woke her up when they arrived, but it was late and Sra. Álvarez was already asleep. Ximena lay in an unfamiliar bed thinking about how effortless the drive had been; no *policía*, no gangs, no hunger or thirst, and no death. She said a prayer for her *familia*'s safety.

"¡*Buenos días!*" Sra. Álvarez knocked on the bedroom door. She was a plump woman with greying hair. "We have a lot of work to do today. We have to go down to school and get you enrolled and go to the store and buy a backpack and school supplies."

"I don't have any money," Ximena said discouraged.

"We are *familia*," she said with a smile.

They drove to a local high school recommended for immigrant students. The school was tiny. They were buzzed in through the front doors and welcomed by a receptionist who handed them a bunch of paperwork. Once they were finished, they waited in the cafeteria. The principal came to greet them within the half-hour, welcoming Ximena to the school's community and handing her the class schedule. Ximena felt overwhelmed.

They returned home and Sra. Álvarez made lunch. Over lunch they talked about what her responsibilities would be around the house, her financial obligations, Sra. Álvarez's academic expectations for Ximena, and Ximena's duty to her *familia*. Ximena was expected to find a job as soon as possible and contribute to living expenses at Sra. Álvarez's house, owing the rest to her *familia* to help pay off the loan. She suggested several local businesses she knew would be safe for Ximena to find work. A local butcher shop was the only place that worked with Ximena's school schedule: she would work from 8:00pm to 4:00am and was to start in 2 weeks' time.

For her young age, Ximena showed a surprising strength of character when telling this part of her story. She was ready to work hard and succeed. After church that Sunday, Ximena spent the better half of the day preparing herself for school the next day. She settled for a pair of jeans and a pink blouse and placed all the new school supplies in her backpack. When her alarm went off in the morning, she jumped out of bed. However, she ended up getting quite lost and arriving to school 20 minutes late. Ximena walked up to the teacher and gave him her pass.

"*Bienvenida*, please take a seat," he said in Spanish. This was the first interaction she had with an American teacher. Did everyone in the U.S. speak Spanish too?

"You're in my seat," She heard. The entire class was staring at her. She felt a tug on her shirt from someone one table over.

"This seat is open." Ximena sat down. "My name is Rosa. What's yours? We can get our lunches together."

Ximena and Rosa sat at one of the wooden picnic benches outside and Rosa introduced her to other students at the table. By the time they got their lunches and sat down they had about 15 minutes to eat. Ximena was shoving pizza in her mouth, stuffing her backpack with her leftover milk and an apple before the next period started. Unfortunately, gym class, which came after lunch, was a reminder of the times Ximena spent playing games with her brothers and sisters. She tried not to think about how much she missed her family. Her grandma got sick, and she knew she could not see her before she passed. At weekends when she wasn't at church, she was cleaning the house.

School became more and more difficult to manage once she started working. Her day consisted of seven hours of school followed by 8 hours of work and 3 hours of homework. Nonetheless, work kept her distracted from her thoughts as she spent her shift cutting meat and cleaning the establishment. At school, some kids had been deported, and it seemed like someone new was missing every month. Ximena ran the risk of being arrested every time she stepped out of the house. Walking to and from school and work became dangerous activities, but at least her *familia* was safe because Ximena wasn't there to make them a target. It took her more than 4 years to graduate and pay off her *familia's* loan. She said that she'd rather work this hard in the U.S. than be murdered.

Crecer muy rápido
Betsy E. Galicia (Translator)

Cuando Bailey entrevistaba a niños no acompañados encontró patrones que se repetían. Por ejemplo, los niños solían empezar a hablar sobre los recuerdos de su familia. Durante la entrevista, Ximena, una joven de 17 años, dijo que crecer. Era la segunda de siete hijos y frecuentemente ayudaba a su mamá con los quehaceres de la casa, que incluían el cuidado de los hermanos menores, así como cocinar y limpiar. Su hermano mayor, Edgar, empezó a trabajar en los cerros con su papá en cuanto cumplió doce años. Cuando se iban a trabajar por semanas o meses. Aunque no veía a su papá o a Edgar por largos periodos de tiempo, cuando regresaban era como si nunca se hubieran ido. Pasaban las noches juntos, cenando, contando historias, o jugando al arranca cebolla[4] o la tripa chuca.[5] Su papá siempre les traía regalos: piedras de todas formas y tamaños, una para cada niño. Ximena tomaba cada piedra y la pulía junto a la quebrada cerca de su casa. Hacía collares de las piedras usando alambres e hilo que encontraba cuando ayudaba a su mamá en la finca. Luego, cuando su hermana tuvo la edad suficiente para cuidar a los cuatro hermanos más pequeños, se le permitió ir con su mamá al mercado. Vendía joyas junto con el maíz, los huevos, y el azúcar que cultivaban en su finca. Le encantaba pasar tiempo con su mamá, pero el verdadero regalo era poder ver la televisión en la tienda con aire acondicionado de la Sra. Rodríguez.

Bailey encontró que el tema de la pobreza surgía frecuentemente en las entrevistas con niñas adolescentes y en particular expresaban el deseo de pertenecer en el mundo de fantasía de la televisión donde el dinero abundaba y se malgastaba. La casa de Ximena no tenía electricidad, así que en la tienda de la Sra. Rodríguez era donde podía ver la tele. Su programa favorito trataba sobre cuatro amigas que iban a la misma escuela. Ximena nunca había ido a la escuela, pero soñaba con ir, usar maquillaje, hablar con los chicos y llevar la ropa de las gringas. Ellas tenían el cabello lindísimo y el maquillaje perfecto y todos los chicos las querían. Un día Ximena derritió la crayola de su hermana pequeña y lo mezcló con aceite para hacerse un lápiz labial para verse igual de bonita que las gringas en la tele. Su mamá olió el crayón derretido y le dio una nalgada por arruinar el único crayón rosa que tenían. Sin embargo, Ximena guardó su creación brillante en una lata debajo de su almohada y planeó estrenarla en su quinceañera, que iba a ser en unas semanas.

Su mamá le hizo un vestido rosa y planearon ir a misa con toda la familia. Hicieron pupusas y pastel, y mandaron las invitaciones a toda la familia. Todo lo que Ximena quería para su quinceañera era un par de zapatos nuevos. Solamente había asistido a una quinceañera antes y era la de su prima Isela. Se acordaba de la tiara que lucía su prima con la que se veía exactamente como una princesa. Su tía le dijo que la peinaría igual que a Isela y que podría tomar prestados sus zapatos para la ceremonia.

Desafortunadamente, otro denominador común en la investigación de Bailey son las memorias del día en que los niños son agredidos. El día de sus quince, el padre de Ximena la llevó al salón para que su tía la peinara. Estaba fresco. Cuando llegaron al salón, su tía le explicó que tenía que terminar con otro cliente. Ximena se sentó afuera y su tía le dijo que no se alejara. Aburrida se paseaba cerca del salón. Le chiflaron un grupo de chicos, sintió miedo y regresó al salón para que su tía la peinara. Cuando terminó, Ximena fue en busca de su padre que la estaba esperando en un bar cercano. De camino al bar, vio al mismo grupo de chicos que le habían chiflado antes y la llamaron. Bajó la cabeza y siguió caminando hacia el bar.

Después de eso, Ximena solo recordaba haber despertado en un cuarto obscuro con sus manos atadas a la espalda y con un dolor punzante en la cabeza. Escuchaba el vaivén de voces inaudibles y empezó a gatear hacia un rayo de luz que salía debajo de la puerta. Unos hombres abrieron la puerta y entraron corriendo. Ximena vio un hombre joven que tenía tatuajes que le cubrían la cara y el cuello. Las uñas de la mano las tenía puntiagudas y filosas y parecían cuernos. Era delgado y llevaba una playera blanca sin mangas. Tenía una pistola en la cintura.

"¡Escribe el número de celular de tus padres!" le gritó mientras le apuntaba con la pistola en la cabeza.

Le dijo que no tenían teléfono, pero él se rio. Le pegó en la sien con la pistola. Ximena sintió que su cabeza se calentaba y empezó a orarle a Dios.

"Vivo cerca de las montañas en una finca" pudo decir entre sollozos.

"Puta madre. Es pobre," dijo el joven.

Ximena estuvo temblando hasta que oyó una voz nueva.

"Dile a tu mamá que estás viva," le ordenó y puso el teléfono en su oído.

"Te amo" fue todo lo que tuvo tiempo de decir.

"Tienes 24 horas para obtener el dinero, si la quiere viva." Colgó el teléfono y se fue.

Su mamá y papá vendieron todo lo que tenían, incluyendo el par de zapatos nuevos que le habían comprado para sus quince. Pidieron prestado a miembros de la familia, pero su respuesta no fue lo suficientemente rápida.

Al siguiente día, a la misma hora, cuatro hombres entraron al cuarto, dejando entrar una luz destellante. Tomaron turnos profanando su cuerpo, violándola, derramándole cerveza, y golpeándola. Ximena empezó a orar y a pensar en su familia tratando de bloquear el miedo.

"¡Tenemos el dinero!" gritó uno de ellos, y poco después, le cubrieron la cabeza con una bolsa, pero ni siquiera se tomaron la molestia de cubrirle su cuerpo desnudo. La cargaron en un auto y la transportaron de regreso al pueblo. El auto apenas frenó lo suficiente y la empujaron hacia afuera. Sus brazos estaban atados y su cabeza seguía cubierta. Ximena se quedó sin moverse en el pavimento. No podía decir cuánto tiempo pasó antes de oír a una mujer gritar al verla.

"Ayúdeme, por favor" le gritó Ximena. La mujer la vistió, le dio comida, y llamó a la policía. La policía llegó en minutos y le hicieron muchas preguntas. Su mente estaba en blanco. Tenía dificultad en recordar cualquier cosa.

La policía la llevó de regreso a su casa. Pasó todo el recorrido intentando recordar algo, cualquier cosa. Cuando salió del coche su familia salió corriendo hacia ella. Entonces recordó el hombre de los tatuajes en la cara y el cuello. Describió a la policía los tatuajes del hombre. Parecía que sabían quién era y ella sintió una oleada de alivio.

Los siguientes dos meses pasaron volando. Su familia estaba a merced de una policía que no tenía poder frente las maras. La policía había encontrado al joven tatuado, pero la mayoría de los días deseaba que no lo hubieran encontrado porque era un miembro de alto rango de La Mara Salvatrucha, conocida como la MS-13. Fue condenado a un mes de cárcel. La MS-13 no sabía dónde vivía, pero se enterarían pronto. El día después de la sentencia, encontraron a la tía de Ximena muerta y la policía reportó que había sido un accidente. El Salvador ya no era lugar seguro para ella. Tenía que irse.

Su familia no tenía los medios financieros para pagar un coyote, así que pidieron dinero prestado otra vez. Le rogó a su papá que le dejara hacer el viaje sin la ayuda de un coyote, pero se marchó a la medianoche con el coyote y su collar de piedras favorito. Su vida estaba ahora en manos de un extraño llamado Miguel, e iban hacia la "tierra de las oportunidades".

La historia de migración de Ximena conllevaba muchos riesgos como ser reconocida por afiliados a la MS13, estar a merced de un guía desconocido, y sobrevivir al agotamiento, el hambre y la sed del viaje. Se unió a un grupo de siete personas guiadas por Miguel. Tomaron un autobús que los llevó hasta un pueblo pequeño en México. Allí fueron detenidos e inspeccionados en México por la policía, quienes les hicieron pagar dinero antes de dejarlos continuar. Miguel les aconsejó que se calmaran durante este tipo de inspecciones, pero Ximena podía sentir que las rodillas le temblaban y que le caía el sudor por la cara. Ya habían viajado por un par de días y estaban racionando las comidas en pequeñas cantidades de pan y agua. Ximena tenía sed y hambre insaciable, pero sabía que tenía que ahorrar el pan para condiciones más duras.

Viajaron por muchos días y noches por el desierto. Tal vez viajaban lentamente, pero lo hacían seguro. Vieron varios cuerpos de personas que habían tratado de hacer el viaje demasiado rápido o se habían encontrado con Los Zetas.[6] El tufo era insoportable y Ximena se encontró ahogándose ante el olor a cadáver podrido por el sol. Se preocupaba por otra viajera, Marta, y su bebé. Se enfermó y se estaba desnutriendo más rápido que el resto del grupo. Ximena compartió su pan con ella. Pero se estaba quedando sin comida y aún quedaba mucho camino por recorrer.

Después de muchos días y noches en el desierto, se había terminado el pan hacía tiempo y el agua era escasa. Ximena desvariaba por momentos. Cuando llegaron al río ya era de noche. El aire estaba húmedo y el agua estaba tranquila. Sabía que una nueva vida la esperaba al otro lado del río, pero no se sentía completamente lista para dejar su vida anterior.

Se amontonaron en balsas y les dijeron que se quedaran callados mientras los hombres remaban. Flotaron lentamente a través del río, sin querer perturbar el flujo natural del agua, ni crear demasiado ruido. El punto de entrada escogido por el coyote estaba cubierto de arbustos. Él ayudó a cada persona a subir a la tierra. Marta fue la primera mientras Ximena sostenía al bebé Kevin. Agarró a Kevin cuidadosamente de las manos de Ximena. Ximena empezó a hacer su ascenso, pero la maleza que estaba utilizando como ancla se desprendió de la tierra. Su pie resbaló y en seguida estaba completamente sumergida en el agua. Rápidamente Miguel agarró la pierna de Ximena y puso su dedo índice verticalmente sobre sus labios. En silencio, estaban oficialmente en los Estados Unidos y cada uno tenía su propio viaje por completar.

El trabajo del coyote ya estaba hecho, y Ximena tenía la tarea de buscar a la prima de su mamá. Con precaución, siguió viajando hacia el norte. Se mantuvo escondida lo más que pudo y rehusó descansar hasta que llegó a un teléfono público. No tenía comida, ni agua, y no había dormido una noche entera en casi dos meses. Estaba sucia y llevaba roba sucia, pero la caída al río le había quitado la mayoría del tufo. Pidió ayuda para encontrar el teléfono público más cercano. Se encontró con una mujer joven que empujaba a su bebé en un cochecito por la acera y ésta le preguntó si le podía ayudar. Sonrió y dijo: "¿teléfono público?" y sacó un celular de su bolsillo, indicándole que lo usara. Ximena marcó el número de teléfono y esperó a que le contestará la prima de su mamá.

"¿Bueno?"

"¿Es la Sra. Álvarez?" La otra persona se calló. "¿Hola? Soy yo, la hija de Mariana." Era como si ella estuviera hablando con un fantasma.

"¿Estás a salvo? ¿Dónde estás?" le preguntó.

La Sra. Álvarez le dio la dirección de una amiga que vivía cerca de donde estaba. Era donde debía quedarse hasta que su hijo viniera a recogerla por la mañana. Mientras iba a la dirección que le dio, se fijó en el paisaje; había muchas iglesias y notó que las marquesinas de madera decían 28 de agosto del 2012. No sabía que el viaje había tomado dos meses; le pareció una eternidad.

"Estoy buscando a la Sra. Huerta. La Sra. Álvarez me mandó," dijo nerviosamente en la entrada. Un hombre la invitó a entrar y llamó a la Sra. Huerta, su esposa. Una mujer mayor de baja estatura salió de la cocina.

"¡Justo a tiempo! ¡He preparado menudo!" Ximena miró al señor que le señaló el camino a la cocina. Llena de alegría a Ximena empezó a llorar. La Sra. Huerta miró a su esposo y le dijo a Ximena "Estás a salvo aquí; buen provecho".

La voz de Ximena se hacía más fuerte en esta parte esperanzadora de su historia.

La Sra. Huerta le dio un atuendo y un par de zapatos. Pasaron la mañana hablando sobre planes para la escuela, hacer amigos, y trabajar para ayudar a pagar el préstamo de sus padres. Alberto llegó al atardecer. Hablaba bien, iba bien vestido y tenía buenos modales. Tenía el automóvil más lindo que Ximena había visto. Estaba tan impresionada por el auto que casi se le olvidó darle las gracias a la Sra. Huerta y a su esposo por su hospitalidad. Se sentó en el asiento delantero y vio todos los botones. Alberto se dio cuenta que estaba hipnotizada por los aparatos desconocidos y se rio.

"Chulo, ¿verdad? Lo acabo de comprar con el dinero que ahorré del trabajo". Ximena quería trabajar donde él trabajaba.

Fue un viaje largo y finalmente se quedó dormida. El la despertó cuando llegaron a su casa, pero la Sra. Álvarez estaba ya durmiendo. Ximena se acostó en una cama pensando en lo fácil que había sido el viaje; sin policía, sin pandillas, sin hambre ni sed y sin muerte. Dijo una oración por la seguridad de su familia.

"¡Buenos días!" La Sra. Álvarez tocó la puerta de la habitación. Era una mujer llenita con el cabello gris. "Tenemos mucho trabajo que hacer hoy. Tenemos que ir a la escuela para matricularte e ir a la tienda y comprarte una mochila y útiles escolares."

"No tengo dinero", le dijo desanimada.

"Somos familia", dijo con una sonrisa.

Condujeron a la escuela local recomendada para estudiantes inmigrantes. La escuela era pequeña. Les dejaron entrar por la puerta principal y las recibió una recepcionista. La Sra. Álvarez explicó por qué estaban ahí y la recepcionista les dio un montón de papeles. En cuanto terminaron de llenarlos, esperaron en la cafetería. El director fue a saludarles al rato, les dio la bienvenida a la comunidad de la escuela, y les dio el horario escolar. Ximena se sintió abrumada.

Regresaron a casa y la Sra. Álvarez preparó el almuerzo. Durante el almuerzo hablaron acerca de cuáles serían sus responsabilidades en la casa, sus obligaciones financieras, las expectativas académicas de la Sra. Álvarez, y su deber hacia su familia. Esperaba que Ximena encontrara trabajo lo más pronto posible y que contribuyera a una parte de los gastos del hogar, mandándole el resto a su familia para que pagaran el préstamo. Ella sugirió varios negocios locales que eran seguros para Ximena. El carnicero era el único negocio que encajaba con su horario escolar. Iría a trabajar de 8:00pm a 4:00am y empezaría en dos semanas.

Por su corta edad, Ximena mostraba una sorprendente fortaleza cuando explicaba esta parte de su historia. Después de la iglesia aquel domingo, Ximena pasó la mayor parte del día tratando de encontrar un atuendo apropiado para la escuela. Se decidió por un par de pantalones y una blusa rosa y puso todos los útiles escolares en la mochila. Cuando sonó la alarma en la mañana, saltó de la cama. Sin embargo, se perdió de camino a la escuela y llegó veinte minutos tarde. Ximena caminó hacia el maestro y le dio el pase.

"Bienvenida, por favor toma un asiento", dijo en español. Era su mi primera interacción con un maestro. "hablaban español?", pensó.

"Estás en mi asiento", escuchó. Toda la clase la observaba. Sintió un tirón en la blusa de alguien en la mesa de al lado.

"Este asiento está libre." Se sentó ahí. "Me llamo Rosa. ¿Cómo te llamas?" Podemos ir por el almuerzo juntas."

Ximena y Rosa se sentaron en uno de los bancos de madera exteriores y le presentó a los demás estudiantes sentados en la mesa. En lo que fueron para sus almuerzos y se sentaron, solo les quedaban quince minutos para comer. Ximena engullía a pizza y guardaba en su mochila la leche y la manzana para estar lista antes de que comenzara el siguiente periodo, la clase de gimnasia. Desafortunadamente, la clase de educación física le recordaba los momentos en que jugaba con sus hermanos. Trataba de no pensar en lo mucho que extrañaba a su familia. Los fines de semana si no estaba en la iglesia, estaba limpiando la casa.

La escuela se hizo más difícil de manejar cuando empezó a trabajar. Un día normal para ella consistía en siete horas de escuela seguidas por ocho horas de trabajo y tres horas de tarea. Sin embargo, el trabajo la mantenía distraída de su nostalgia mientras pasaba su turno cortando carne y limpiando el local. En la escuela, algunos niños habían sido deportados y parecía que cada mes faltaba alguien. Corría el riesgo de ser arrestada cada vez que salía de la casa. Caminar de ida y vuelta de la escuela y del trabajo se había convertido en una actividad peligrosa, pero por lo menos su familia estaba a salvo porque Ximena no estaba allí para convertirlos en objetivo de las maras. Le tomó cuatro años graduarse y pagar el préstamo familiar. Dijo que prefería trabajar así de duro en los Estados Unidos a ser asesinada.

Notes

1. Loosely translated "uproot the onion" is a game played by children during which one child grabs a base, such as a tree, and each additional child creates a chain by grabbing hold of the waist of the child in front of them. The children then try to pull those in front of them to pull the first child from the base.
2. Loosely translated "dirty intestines" is a game played with a writing utensil and paper. Pairs of numbers are written in random places on the paper. The object of the game is to connect each number with its pair without touching the lines drawn between other pairs.
3. A powerful crime organization originating in Los Angeles, California.
4. Aproximadamente traducido de "desarraigar la cebolla", este es un juego jugado por niños durante el cual un niño toma una base, como un árbol, y cada niño adicional crea una cadena agarrando la cintura del niño frente a ellos. Luego, los niños tratan de sacar a los que están frente a ellos para sacar al primer niño de la base.

5. Aproximadamente traducido a "intestinos sucios", este es un juego jugado con un utensilio de escribir y papel. Los pares de números se escriben en lugares al azar en el papel. El objetivo del juego es conectar cada número con su par sin tocar las líneas trazadas entre los otros pares.

6. Una poderosa organización criminal originaria de Los Ángeles, California.

Part II

MEMORIES AND BONDS

MELISSA BRIONES, ALFONSO MERCADO, ABIGAIL NUNEZ-SAENZ, PAOLA QUIJANO, AND ANDY TORRES

The story of Salvadorian Toñito depicts the love between a migrant son and his young mother as a symbol for the love and solidarity among migrants in respite centers. The power of a smile is the narrative thread of this story, a healing human connection that often writers experience at the humanitarian center. Although the time they spent with migrants it is only a step of their journeys, the stories they share leave a lasting footprint on the hearts of this Texas community, its volunteers, student research assistants, and Dr. Mercado.

Buscando un destino[1]

Toñito looks out the bus window and sees a girl holding her parents' hands. He can imagine the sound of her laughter as she throws her head back. Her parents smile affectionately down at her. His mother hasn't smiled at him since they met Mr. Jacinto in Mexico. The man they call "*El Coyote*." The *migra* agent calls out in choppy Spanish that this is where we're getting off. He tells Toñito's mom that the bus station is across the street. They are to get on buses and await their immigration court date. His mom holds a packet of papers with her. Toñito tried peaking at them; one of them has a weird title, "Removal Proceedings." He looks up at his mom and smiles. *Ella no sonríe.*

He takes his first free steps on United States ground—where he will finally walk around without having every move watched. Cars zoom by and people stroll holding *papitas* or *paletas*. Toñito's stomach grumbles as he watches a chip fall onto the grimy street.

A man approaches them in Spanish. He leads them to a respite center where he says they will help them. As they walk into the humble building, everyone inside claps. There are the first smiles he has seen in weeks. The people who work there explain the different stations available to get clothes, food, and toiletries. The mention of food piques Toñito's excitement.

He tugs at his *Mamá's* sleeve and she looks down at him. "*¿Qué quieres Toñito?*"

"*Mami, ¡aquí si nos van a dar de comer!*" He tells her excitedly.

Before they can get food or clothes, they have to sign in with the older ladies in the front.

"*¡Hola! Me llamo Sylvia. ¿Cómo se llaman ustedes? ¿Son hermanitos?*"

"*No, él es mi hijo Toñito. Antonio Hernández Mejía. Y yo me llamo Marta Hernández Mejía, para servirle.*"

"*Bueno, Marta. Mucho gusto en conocerlos. ¿A dónde van?*"

The people around them have large yellow envelopes with bus tickets to their next stop. Marta looks down at the tracker clasped around her ankle and murmurs, "*Aún seguimos sin destino.*" Marta would sometimes place a sweater or a bag on her leg to cover the thing on her ankle—the government thing that tracked her everywhere she went.

Sylvia tightens her lips in a sympathetic smile. "*Bueno Marta, primero coman y descansen. Al rato les ayudamos.*"

They shuffle to the next station: toiletries. They get shampoo, soap, toothbrushes, and toothpaste. How amazing would this have been on their journey? Toñito remembers when *Mamá* used to nag him to brush his teeth. Now, he wanted nothing more. The man at the toiletry station put everything in a backpack and told them to have a seat at one of the tables to eat. Toñito didn't have to be told twice. A young volunteer looked for clean clothes for them while they ate chicken noodle soup. Their clothes were stiff from the river water they crossed through. Toñito happily rolled the corn tortilla into a tight roll between his palms like his mom taught him before leaving *abuela's* house in El Salvador. He dipped the rolled tortilla into the broth of his soup and sighed contentedly at the warm trail it left in his throat.

Next, they headed to the outdoor showers. Toñito giggled as *Mamá* made bubbles with the shampoo in his hair. The cool water soothed his small, tired body. He looked at his mother's pretty face and noticed the bags under her eyes that only seemed to get deeper as the days on their journey elapsed. Her face looked thinner and bonier, too.

"*¿Mami, estás bien?*" He asked.

"*Sí, Toñito. Ya van a mejorar las cosas.*"

It was past midnight when his mother began to breathe heavily in a frantic manner. She cried. Toñito wriggled closer and put his arms around her, but she shrugged him away.

"*¡Suéltame! ¡Suéltame, maldito!*" Her voice pierced the night. She wouldn't wake up. The other families in the tent began to stir and groan at the commotion.

"*¡Mamá, mamá! ¡Despierta! ¡Soy yo, Toñito!*" A crown of sweat formed around her head on the pillow. Her hair was wet with tears. The security guard came into the tent flashing his light.

"*Señora. Señora. Despierte,*" the guard said. She breathed in deeply as if she had been drowning. She looked around disoriented until she saw Toñito and pulled him against her shaking body.

"Ay, *Toñito,*" she whispered to him between bouts of sobs. She fingered the rosary she wore on her neck, and they began to pray and praying soothed her. It was the best sleep Toñito had had since leaving El Salvador.

In the morning, they got sweet bread and hot chocolate for breakfast. *Mamá* was starting to look a lot better. Toñito saw a little girl carrying a stuffed bunny. Toñito missed his toy car. But just like *abuela*, they were left behind in El Salvador.

"*¡Mamá, voy a ver los juguetes!*"

"*Mijo, no sé si necesitas permiso.*"

"*No se necesita permiso, puede ir a jugar,*" said one of the volunteers in a blue vest.

"*¡Puedo ir mamá! ¡Por favor!*"

"*Bueno, pero te me portas bien.*"

Toñito ran to the playpen. The toys took him to another world. A world with friends; a world without people shouting: "Go back to where you came from!" He saw a blue racecar and imagined driving it through the streets singing along to the *reggaetón*.

"*Oye, ¿puedo jugar contigo?*" Children aligned colors and rulers to make the track.

"*¿Listos? Cada quien va agarrar un carro y el que llega primero gana.*"

"*Bueno. Yo cuento. 1 ... 2 ... 3 ...*"

"*Gané.*"

"*¡Otra, otra, otra!*" Everyone chanted.

"*¡Venga Ricardo, tú puedes!*" Shouted his mom.

"I bet you guys can't beat me! *¡A mí no me ganan!*" exclaimed the guy who had driven them to this Respite Center. "*A ver todos: ¡el que pierda le toca barrer!*"

Marta was quiet and shy, but she was smiling for the first time in what seemed like forever.

"*¡Dale, Toñito!*" his mom encouraged him.

"*¿Puedo jugar?*" a girl asked as she held her mom's hand. She had a toy car in her hands.

"*¡Claro!*" Toñito answered.

"*Si yo gano me das tu jugo. Y si gano yo, hago la próxima pista.*" The room was buzzing with excitement.

Toñito had newly found friends and his mother was smiling. The respite center wasn't their home, but it felt like it. For the first time in weeks, Toñito heard his mom laugh.

"*Uno, dos, dos y tres cuartos, y . . . y . . . tres!*"

"*¡Vamos Ricardo! ¡Venga Toñito! ¡Vamos hijo! ¡Gánales mijo!*"

The children didn't care who won, because they liked hearing their names being yelled without meaning harm.

"*¿Señora Marta Hernández Mejía?*" a volunteer called.

"*Sí, soy yo,*" she said apprehensively.

"*Tranquila, solo quisiera que platiquemos sobre su destino. Toñito se puede quedar allí. Venga conmigo acá a la mesa en frente.*" The lady and Toñito's mom sat. "*Bueno cuénteme, ¿adónde va? ¿Quién la recibe en los Estados Unidos?*"

"*No sé a dónde voy. Mi tío me dijo que aquí ya no sufriría. Que aquí mi hijo podría ir a la escuela y que ya no nos amenazarían de muerte. El quedó de comprar los boletos una vez que llegáramos aquí. Pero no me contesta y no sé dónde vive en California.*" Marta placed her tired face in her hands. "*Ay, ya no sé qué hacer. Me advirtieron que si no presto a mijo para que distribuya allá con las pandillas me lo van a matar. Y si él no me contesta vamos a tener que regresar.*" There was a pause that consumed time and hope. "*Él es mi vida.*"

"*Mire, es importante que se presente con el juez. Entréguele estos papeles una vez que llegue a la corte. Es una orden para presentarse ante la corte.*"

"*Pero disculpe, ¿cómo puede ser eso? ¿Alguien me puede explicar?*" Marta panicked.

"*No tenga miedo. Lo importante es que usted se presente con el juez. Usted como el resto de las familias, tiene una orden de presentarse ante la corte. El juez determinará su caso, dependiendo de la razón de venir a los Estados Unidos. Doña, es importante que vaya con el juez. Lo último que queremos es que vengan por usted y su hijo. No la quiero espantar. Solo la informo. Si usted tiene preguntas háganos saber. Aquí estamos para usted y Toñito.*" The lady tried to calm her down.

Los días pasaron volando. Before they knew it, they had spent a week at the center. Toñito wore one of the green vests and helped other people. He clapped when newcomers arrived with the other volunteers. "*¡Bienvenidos!*" Toñito guided them through the stations, helped them find clothes, and got them anything else they needed. Once a student from college came by and taught Toñito the names of all the states. She even made a song out of it and had everyone sing it. Toñito dreamt about going to school. His mother would be so proud. He was happy to be walking with her around the respite center under the sun. Some evenings he would play *fútbol* with the other kids while Marta helped the volunteers cook the *sopa*. You could hear them chatting and laughing from far away with a cacophony of clanks from the pots and dishes. Those evenings were the best. His mother wouldn't cry. That's how Toñito knew the days were good. *Pero como dice Mamá, todo lo bueno se acaba.*

Toñito was in the playpen when *Mamá* yelled for him. He saw her crying.

"*¿Que pasó, Mamá?*" he asked.

"*Toñito, aún se nos complican las cosas, hijo,*" she said. "*Tío ha fallecido. Ay, Toñito. Ahora no sé qué va pasar con nosotros.*"

"*¿Y tía, Mamá?*"

"*No la conozco muy bien. Pero como quiera voy a intentar hablar con ella para ver si nos echa una mano.*"

Esa misma noche she prayed all night. *Su carita* was covered in tears. Every now and then she would get close to Toñito and kiss his forehead, but he pretended to be asleep. All Toñito wanted was for his mom to smile and to be drinking *chocolatito caliente en el cantón como antes.*

The next day, Toñito packed the little he had and sadly got ready to leave this *destino* filled with happiness and fun behind. *Y pues como decía mi abuela, se le acabó el dulce al chicle.*

Nuevo destino: Los Angeles, California.

The trip was long and confusing. Because they couldn't speak English, they almost missed their bus. Toñito wanted to learn English—so that he could take his mom around the world one day. He imagined walking with

Mamá in a giant city park full of snow, like the one in the book at the playpen.

"Your ID please?" A man in a green uniform asked them. Toñito's mom said nothing and handed over the paperwork in the yellow envelope that the people at the respite center had given to her.

"What's your name? Is he your little brother?" He asked.

Marta was nervous but was able to answer all the questions they had once they brought a translator. The holster on his waist scared her as much as it scared Toñito. They had spent nights shivering next to each other, days struggling to find food and water, and moments in which neither of them knew where to go next. *A pesar de todo eso*, their *cariño* kept them strong, but now they were afraid. They had fled from armed men just to find more here. *Mamá* held Toñito by his shoulders.

"*Hay que ser fuertes hijo, ya casi llegamos.*" She whispered.

"*La migra chequea que todos en el bus traigan papeles. Siempre hacen eso cerca de la frontera. A mí me tocó que me checaran allá en Tejas. En ese entonces solo tenía la visa. Me dio miedo . . .*" a woman said to her friend once the man got off the bus.

A la noche siguiente, the bus stopped at the bus station. Toñito kept looking out the window hoping to see the *tío*. He thought of what his mom had said: he had a beard and that he always wore brown boots and . . . but Toñito remembered tío *ya no está con nosotros*. He had forgotten.

"*Vámonos, hijo. Creo que tía ya nos espera. Apúrate, hijo mío.*" *Mamá* rushed him out of the bus as she gripped his hand tighter.

"*¿Como la vamos a encontrar?*" Toñito asked.

"*Ponte el suéter, te vas a enfermar, el autobús estaba caliente . . .*"

"*Ma, no tengo frío.*"

"*No desobedezcas, está frío y yo no sé qué haría si te me enfermas. PÓN-TELO.*"

"*¡Ma! ¡No!*"

"*Que te lo pongas, no me hagas volver a decirte, estamos en público, ten prudencia Toñito. Póntelo.*"

"*¡ANTONIO!*" They both turned towards the voice that shouted his name.

"*Tú debes ser Antonio,*" a woman said.

"*Ay tía Rosa disculpe, mire lo siento, muchas gracias por todo se lo agradezco con toda la fuerza del cielo—*"

"*Vámonos, niña.*" The lady cut her off.

Rosa's stare was cold, and she kept her hands in the pockets of her jacket. Toñito saw her black hair dangling on her back covering a scar on the back of her neck. She walked fast. She didn't talk or even look at us. She kept ignoring his mother's attempts to thank her, which both frustrated and worried Toñito.

"*Antonio, ya. Póntelo.*" she told me again as she spread her arms to put my jacket over my shoulders.

"*No, póntelo tú.*"

Slap!

Rosa's handprint on Toñito's cheek stung. Rosa kept talking but all Toñito could hear was his mother's fingers on her rosary as she prayed. Toñito could hear his mom's heartbeat and she could feel his tears over her sweater.

¿Y si nos secuestra? ¿Y si ella lastima a mamá? ¿Y si nos pierde porque no nos quiere? ¿Y si tenemos que vivir en la calle porque ella nos corre? ¿Por qué nos pasa esto? Yo solo quería que mamá no llorase tanto y que nadie nos lastime pero venimos a lo mismo aquí. Ya no quiero estar aquí—

"*¡Mijo, Mijo, MIJO, vámonos!*" *Mamá* shook Toñito by the shoulder. "*Ay Toñito, estás bañado en sudor, ojalá no te me vayas a resfriar,*" she whispered.

Toñito wanted to tell her that he was scared. He wanted to tell her that his legs were still shaking and that he could hear his own heart jumping. He wanted to tell her that he wished we were back on the ranch with grandma. He wanted to tell her that he wanted to be eating *pupusas de queso* with the family. That he wanted to go back in time like Superman to when she would tuck him in bed with a prayer and a kiss on the forehead. He wanted to say all these things to her, but he kept silent.

Toñito started having nightmares, but one kept going on through daytime. *Mamá* would wake up every morning at 4 AM to cook Rosa's lunch for work. She would then wash and dry everyone's clothes. After lunch and before 1 o'clock, she was back to cleaning. She would grab the broom and mop and clean the entire house. Even though she was always in a rush, she usually finished just in time to cook something for Rosa. If by 6 PM dinner was not ready, Rosa would get angry. By 7 PM, she had to clean and wash dishes again and start getting ready for the next day. She had Toñito saying the good night prayer every time. Sometimes she would fall asleep from exhaustion before Toñito was done praying.

The best days were Sundays. Rosa didn't wake up until noon, so they would wake up when the sky was still dark and walk to church to hear the earliest mass. It was the only hour of the week when Toñito saw *Mamá* at peace. They listened to the priest and sang all of the songs. They didn't have any money for the *ofrenda*, but his mom always said that *Diosito* would understand. After church, they would take a walk to a nearby park. She would push Toñito on the swings and let him run around and play. Around 11, they would make their way back to Rosa's house. Toñito was always sad on the way back.

Toñito wanted to know why his mom sometimes had bruises on her arms. They were small and less frequent at first, *pero ahora había muchos, estaban grandes y de diferentes colores. Mamá me decía que se tropezaba y se pegaba limpiando.*

Toñito wanted to know why he couldn't join the rest of the children on the yellow bus every weekday.

"*Algún día cuando seas grande te explicaré mijo,*" she would always say.

On the days that Toñito was really bored, he began to stare out the window. He would count the cars that would go by and watch the other children playing outside. The boy next door would get home in the yellow bus and an hour later he would come out with a soccer ball.

The first time that he saw Toñito looking at him through the window, Toñito pulled the curtains and ran away. The next day when he went outside to play, Toñito peeked through a small open sliver in the curtains. The boy kept looking at the window.

A couple of days passed before Toñito got bored enough to open the curtain again. The boy waved. He waved back. Toñito wasn't allowed to go outside, but he really wanted to go play with the ball. *Él tenía una pelota justo como esa en El Salvador.*

His mom was still out doing the laundry. She wouldn't be back for another hour. If Toñito went outside now, his mom wouldn't notice, so he ran out the door.

"*Hola, me llamo Toñito. ¿Puedo jugar fútbol contigo?*" He asked the boy.

"Hi, Toñito. I'm Marcos. I don't have a football, but we can play with my soccer ball," he replied.

Toñito didn't understand what he said. He spoke fast, but he said *fútbol.* So he moved his feet, and he stole the ball that was secured under his foot.

"Hey, come back!" He yelled. He started running after Toñito.

Toñito made it close to the trash cans and kicked and aimed the ball between them. When the ball went through, he jumped and screamed: "¡GOOOOL!" *Ya hacía mucho tiempo que no jugaba a fútbol. Se me había olvidado la emoción del deporte y qué divertido era.*

"That was an awesome shot!" Marcos said as he high fived Toñito. The boys took turns taking shots at the trash cans, being goalies, and kicking the ball to each other. They had so much fun, but Toñito needed to get back inside soon before his mom got home.

"*Una más*," Toñito raised one finger. "*Me tengo que regresar a mi casa*," He pointed at the house. Marcos nodded and began running toward the trash cans where Toñito was holding guard. After the game was over, Toñito ran home just before his mom got there.

Marcos's friendship made the days go by faster and life a lot sweeter. It was all going well until *that* day.

Marcos got near and kicked the ball. He tried to grab the ball in midair, but it hit Toñito straight in the face.

"Ahh!" Toñito screamed, with a burning sensation on his face.

Marcos ran toward him. "Are you okay? I'm so sorry. I didn't mean to hit your head. Can you stand up?"

Me duele mucho la cabeza. No me puedo levantar. Me siento mareado. He saw Marcos run away. "*¿Adónde vas?*" He tried to yell, but it came out like a soft whisper.

Toñito tried to get up, but he felt disoriented and lost. It hurt so much. He couldn't open his eyes. He heard footsteps. "Are you okay?" A soft, melodic voice asked.

Toñito couldn't reply. "Mom, he doesn't speak English," said Marcos.

Toñito worried about what his mom would think, he knew she would be upset.

"Marcos, please grab another chair for Toñito's mom," Toñito opened his eyes slowly, feeling pressure and pain in his head. Toñito couldn't get up. He felt nauseous.

"Toñito is going to be … *va estar bien señora. Siéntese. ¿Quiere un* coffee … *café?*"

"*¿Seguro que va estar bien señora? ¿Qué le pasó? Yo lo dejé dentro de la casa. Siempre le digo que no se salga porque le puede pasar algo y no conocemos a nadie aquí …*" Her voice trailed off.

"*Sí, va estar bien. Me dijo Marcos que pateó la pelota y accidentalmente le pegó a Toñito en la cabeza. Yo soy una enfermera. Si se siente muy mal lo llevamos al doctor.*" There was her melodic voice.

"*Yo no tengo dinero para ir a un doctor,*" his mom said softly.

"*No se preocupe, ¿cómo se llama?*"

"*Marta y ¿usted?*"

"*Yo me llamo Hope, o en español, Esperanza.*"

"*Qué hermoso nombre.*"

"*Gracias, Marta. Mire, su hijo va estar bien. Nada más fue un golpe. No le pasó nada y aquí va a estar bien.*" Hope reassured her. "*¿Va a querer un café?*"

"*Sí, muchas gracias.*"

"*Bueno. Déjeme traerle el café . . . ¿de dónde es usted? Se le oye el* accent *muy diferente,*" said Hope as she whipped up a coffee.

"*Nosotros somos de El Salvador.*"

"Wow, *qué lejos. ¿Está bonito allá? Mis papás son de Colombia.*"

"*Mi país es hermoso pero la violencia lo ha echado a perder. Hay demasiada violencia y uno no puede vivir cómodo. Ya iban unos años que vivimos bajo las sombras porque las pandillas andan donde quiera.*"

"How scary . . . *qué miedo. ¿Es por eso por lo que están aquí en los Estados Unidos?*" She asked amidst the clinking sound of the coffee cups being set on the table.

"*Estamos aquí por muchas razones,*" his mamá said slowly sipping her coffee.

"*Está bien. ¿Cómo les han gustado los Estados? Hay muchos lugares muy bonitos aquí.*"

"*No tenemos mucho dinero. Le limpio la casa y le cocino a la esposa de mi tío. No tenemos mucho tiempo para salir.*"

"*¿Y le pagan a usted por limpiar la casa?*"

"*Mmm no, pero estoy muy agradecida con mi tía. Y es lo único que pide por dejarnos quedar en su casa gratis.*"

"*¿Y tienes otro trabajo?*" she asked.

"*Ahorita no tengo trabajo. No se hablar inglés y pues no tengo tiempo con las tareas domésticas de mi tía. Y también no quiero dejar a Toñito solo por mucho tiempo.*"

"*Ah la entiendo. Yo también no me gusta dejar a mi Marcos solo. Y ahora que ya me separé de mi esposo, se me hace más difícil ir al* work *en las noches.*"

"*¿Lo deja al niño solo en las noches?*"

"*No aquí lo dejo en casa de mi mamá, pero mi mamá también ya está mayor y pues no me gusta dejarlos solos a los dos.*"

Toñito started to feel a little better. He sat up. "*¿Mamá?*" he croaked.

"*Ay Toñito, ¿cómo te sientes? ¿Te duele mucho la cabeza? Me pegaste un susto mi niño.*" Mamá ran toward him.

"*Me duele mucho la cabeza, pero ya me siento un poco mejor.*"

"*Señora Hope, muchas gracias por toda su ayuda. No sé cómo podré pagarle todo lo que ha hecho. Yo y Toñito ya nos tenemos que regresar a la casa de mi tía.*"

"*No se preocupe, Marta. Las puertas de mi casa y las de mi mamá siempre estarán abiertas para ustedes.*"

"*Muchas gracias, Hope.*"

They trudged their way back to Tia Rosa's house dreading what awaited them.

"*¿Dónde has estado niña estúpida? ¡Mal agradecida! No te pido mucho para todo lo que hago por ti y ese niño. Yo no tenía por qué aceptarlos en mi casa. ¡Ni los conozco!*" Rosa yelled at Marta and smacked her cheek, which resonated louder than her voice.

"*Señora Marta, ¿qué sucede?!*" Hope and Marcos stood outside watching Rosa.

"*Lo que pasa es que esta malcriada no tuvo la cena para mí cuando llegué a la casa. ¿Quién sabe dónde estuvo metida esta desgraciada, o más bien con quién estuvo? ¿Verdad? Sinvergüenza.*"

Slap! Rosa's hand landed on Marta's face again.

Suddenly, Hope was at my mother's side. "*¡Señora!* You have no right! *Ella estuvo conmigo. Su hijo no estaba muy bien y lo estaba cuidando.*"

"*Ah, ¿sí? Bueno pues entonces esta niña y su hijo ya no son mi problema. Agarren sus cosas y lárguense de mi vista.*"

Marta sobbed uncontrollably shouting in between breaths, "*¡Ay Dios mío!*" *Y suspirando dijo*, "*¿Qué vamos a hacer ahora?*"

"*Marta y Toñito se vienen conmigo.*"

"*Vámonos mijo, vente,*" *Mamá le dijo entre lágrimas.*

When Toñito woke up, *Mamá* told him to go to the car. He saw Marcos throwing bags of snacks and waters into the backseat of the car. Hope was in the driver's seat. He held his mother's hand tight.

"Tony?" Hope called out. No one had ever called Toñito by that name, but he liked it. "*No se me agite, todo va estar bien.*"

Sometimes family is who you want them to be and not who happens to be.

"*Tome, se va a poner frío*" Hope took her jacket and gave it to his mom.

"*No, como cree, yo estoy bien,*" Marta replied in a broken voice.

"*Tiene que ser fuerte, por usted y Tony.*" Hope *les seguía intentando de calmar.*

"*¡No los dejaremos solos; vámonos, Marcos!*" *dijo* Hope *con una sonrisa.*

The drive was beautiful. Toñito cleaned the tears from his mom's face and kissed her forehead. She prayed next to him, and Toñito felt her warmth cover his face as he fell asleep on her.

"*Mijo, es aquí. Ya llegamos,*" *Mamá* whispered to him.

There was no sun in the sky but there were lights all over the small yet pretty house. *Luces de navidad.* The moment Toñito got out the car he felt a cool breeze on his face. His mom came from behind screaming . . .

"*¡Mijo, somos libres ya!*"

"*¡Bienvenidos!*" Hope screamed with joy.

"I forgot to give you this," Marcos handed Toñito a backpack with one, diagonal strap. "You're going to need it when you go to school with me."

"*Vas ir a la escuela con Marcos, Tony.*" said Hope.

"*¿Iré a la escuela contigo?*" Toñito jumped with excitement. "*¡Ma, Ma! ¿Iré a la escuela con Marcos?*"

Mamá smiled at him.

"*Sí Toñito, irás a la escuela con Marcos. Te podemos hacer* register *la próxima semana. Pero ahora tenemos mucho que hacer. Ahora, ¿quién tiene hambre?* Who's hungry?" Hope asked. Everyone said *yo.* Everyone ran inside the blue house, their new home. At the door, there was sign that read "dream."

From that day on, they lived in a home and not just in a house. Having Hope and Marcos with them was always joyful and safe. Marta took care of Marcos at night when Hope had the night shift at the hospital. Hope also got Toñito's mom a cleaning job at the hospital and she was able to make a good living for them. From that day on, Toñito no longer saw *moretones* on her. And other than for the times she would cut onions for the soup, she no longer cried. The years in school flew by. After a couple of months in a creative writing club in high school, Toñito began writing stories for competitions and even got to travel to other places to compete with other children from schools from all over the country.

In college, Toñito decided to pursue writing. He found solace in writing. Although there was misery and sadness in his journey to the United States, the bliss of seeing his mother so proud of him walking across the stage on his graduation day was worth it.

They still saw Marcos and Hope on occasions. Hope was offered a better job in San Francisco. It was an offer she couldn't refuse. They kept in contact and made sure to reunite at least once a year.

Toñito and his mother were granted Refugee status, which allowed them to stay in the United States. It was a difficult process; both legally and emotionally. His mom explained what *asalto físico* and rape meant and how she had been a victim of both many times. His mom also had to explain that they had been threatened in El Salvador. If they went back, they were sure to meet their deaths. That day Toñito sat next to her in silence, listening to the sound of her heart. Eventually, they were granted Legal Permanent Resident status. They celebrated that day, cherishing the opportunity to stay in this country. There's a beautiful, joyful glint in his mother's eyes. Together, they smile at their found *destino*.[2]

Looking for a Destino[3]

Toñito looks out the bus window and sees a girl holding her parents' hands. He can imagine the sound of her laughter as she throws her head back. Her parents smile affectionately down at her. His mother hasn't smiled at him since they met Mr. Jacinto in Mexico. The man they call "The Smuggler." The border patrol agent calls out in choppy Spanish that this is where we're getting off. He tells Toñito's mom that the bus station is across the street. They are to get on buses and await their immigration court date. His mom holds a packet of papers with her. Toñito tried peaking at them; one of them has a weird title, "Removal Proceedings." He looks up at his mom and smiles. She doesn't smile back at me.

He takes his first free steps on United States ground—where he will finally walk around without having every move watched. Cars zoom by and people stroll holding chips or ice cream pops. Toñito's stomach grumbles as he watches a chip fall onto the grimy street.

A man approaches them in Spanish. He leads them to a respite center where he says they will help them. As they walk into the humble building, everyone inside claps. There are the first smiles he has seen in weeks. The people who work there explain the different stations available to get clothes, food, and toiletries. The mention of food piques Toñito's excitement.

He tugs at his mom's sleeve, and she looks down at him. "¿What do you want, Toñito?"

"Mommy, they're going to feed us here!" He tells her excitedly.

Before they can get food or clothes, they have to sign in with the older ladies in the front.

"Hi. My name is Sylvia. What are your names? Are you brother and sister?"

"No, he is my son Toñito. Antonio Hernandez Mejia. And my name is Marta Hernandez Mejia, at your service."

"Okay, Marta. Very nice to meet you. Where are you going?"

The people around them have large yellow envelopes with bus tickets to their next stop. Marta looks down at the tracker clasped around her ankle and murmurs, "We still don't have a destination." Marta would sometimes place a sweater or a bag on her leg to cover the thing on her ankle—the government thing that tracked her everywhere she went.

Sylvia tightens her lips in a sympathetic smile. "Okay, Marta. First, rest and have a meal. We will help you after."

They shuffle to the next station: toiletries. They get shampoo, soap, toothbrushes, and toothpaste. How amazing would this have been on their journey? Toñito remembers when his mom used to nag him to brush his teeth. Now, he wanted nothing more. The man at the toiletry station put everything in a backpack and told them to have a seat at one of the tables to eat. Toñito didn't have to be told twice. A young volunteer looked for clean clothes for them while they ate chicken noodle soup. Their clothes were stiff from the river water they crossed through. Toñito happily rolled the corn tortilla into a tight roll between his palms like his mom taught him before leaving grandma's house in El Salvador. He dipped the rolled tortilla into the broth of his soup and sighed contentedly at the warm trail it left in his throat.

Next, they headed to the outdoor showers. Toñito giggled as his mom made bubbles with the shampoo in his hair. The cool water soothed his small, tired body. He looked at his mother's pretty face and noticed the bags under her eyes that only seemed to get deeper as the days on their journey elapsed. Her face looked thinner and bonier, too.

"Mommy, are you okay?" He asked.

"Yes, Toñito. Things are going to get better."

It was past midnight when his mother began to breathe heavily in a frantic manner. She cried. Toñito wriggled closer and put his arms around her, but she shrugged him away.

"Let me go! Let me go, you bastard!" Her voice pierced the night. She wouldn't wake up. The other families in the tent began to stir and groan at the commotion.

"Mom, mom! Wake up! It's me! Toñito!" A crown of sweat formed around her head on the pillow. Her hair was wet with tears. The security guard came into the tent flashing his light.

"Miss. Miss. Wake up!" the guard said. She breathed in deeply as if she had been drowning. She looked around disoriented until she saw Toñito and pulled him against her shaking body.

"Oh, Toñito," she whispered to him between bouts of sobs. She fingered the rosary she wore on her neck, and they began to pray and praying soothed her. It was the best sleep Toñito had had since leaving El Salvador.

In the morning, they got sweet bread and hot chocolate for breakfast. His mom was starting to look a lot better. Toñito saw a little girl carrying a stuffed bunny. Toñito missed his toy car. But just like grandma, they were left behind in El Salvador.

"Mom, I'm going to see the toys!"

"Son, I don't know if you need special permission to go."

"No need to ask permission, he can go play," said one of the volunteers in a blue vest.

"Can I go, mom? Please!"

"Fine. But you better behave."

Toñito ran to the playpen. The toys took him to another world. A world with friends; a world without people shouting: "Go back to where you came from!" He saw a blue racecar and imagined driving it through the streets singing along to the reggaeton.

"Hey, can I play with you?" Children aligned colors and rulers to make the track.

"Everyone ready? Each one of us is going to get a car and whoever gets to the finish line first wins."

"Okay. I'll count. 1 . . . 2 . . . 3 . . ."

I won.

"Another one!" Everyone chanted.

"Let's go, Ricardo! You can do it!" Shouted his mom.

"I bet you guys can't beat me! You won't beat me!" exclaimed the guy who had driven them to this Respite Center. "Okay, everybody! Whoever loses has to sweep the whole room!"

Marta was quiet and shy, but she was smiling for the first time in what seemed like forever.

"Go, Toñito!" his mom encouraged him.

"Can I play?" a girl asked as she held her mom's hand. She had a toy car in her hands.

"Of course!" Toñito answered.

"If I win you give me your juice. And if I win, I make the next racetrack." The room was buzzing with excitement.

Toñito had newly-found friends and his mother was smiling. The respite center wasn't their home, but it felt like it. For the first time in weeks, Toñito heard his mom laugh.

"One . . . two . . . two and three quarters . . . and . . . and . . . three!"

Let's go Ricardo! Come on Toñito! Go son! Beat them, son!"

The children didn't care who won, because they liked hearing their names being yelled without meaning harm.

"Miss Marta Hernández Mejía?" a volunteer called.

"Yes, that's me," she said apprehensively.

"No need to worry. I only want to talk about where you are going. Toñito can stay here and keep playing. Come with me to the table in the front," The lady and Toñito's mom sat. "Okay, so tell me. Where are you going? Who is expecting and hosting you in the United States?"

"I'm not sure where I'm going. My uncle told me that I wouldn't suffer here anymore. He said my kid could go to school and we wouldn't be threatened to be killed anymore. He said he would buy the tickets once we were here, but he won't answer his calls and I'm not sure where he lives in California." Marta placed her tired face in her hands. "Ay, I no longer know what to do. I was threatened that if I didn't allow my son to help the gangs distribute (illicit drugs) they would kill him. And if he doesn't answer we will have to go back." There was a pause that consumed time and hope. "He is my life."

"Look, is important that you appear before the judge. Turn in these documents once you arrive at court. This is a Notice to Appear in court."

"But excuse me, how can this be? Can someone explain this to me?" Marta panicked.

"Don't be afraid. What matters is that you appear before the judge. You, like many of the other families, have this order to appear in court (Notice to Appear). The judge will determine your case, depending on your reason of coming to the United Sates. Madam, it is important that you do appear in court. The last thing we want is for them (ICE) to come for you and your son. I don't mean to scare you, just inform you. If you have any questions, please let us know. We are here for you and Toñito." The lady tried to calm her down.

The days flew past. Before they knew it, they had spent a week at the center. Toñito wore one of the green vests and helped other people. He clapped when newcomers arrived with the other volunteers. Welcome! Toñito guided them through the stations, helped them find clothes, and got them anything else they needed. Once a student from college came by and taught Toñito the names of all the states. She even made a song out of it and had everyone sing it. Toñito dreamt about going to school. His mother would be so proud. He was happy to be walking with her around the respite center under the sun. Some evenings he would play soccer with the other kids while mom helped the volunteers cook the soup. You could hear them chatting and laughing from far away with a cacophony of clanks from the pots and dishes. Those evenings were the best. His mother wouldn't cry. That's how Toñito knew the days were good. But as mom says, everything good comes to an end.

Toñito was in the playpen when Mom yelled for him. He saw her crying. "What happened, mom?" he asked.

"Toñito, things have become more complicated, son," she said. "My uncle has died." "Ay, Toñito. Now I don't know what is going to happen to us."

"And your aunt, mom?"

"I don't know her very well. I've heard that she's not as a nice of a person that my uncle was. But I'm still going to try to talk to her tomorrow and see if she can help us out."

That same night she prayed all night. Her face was covered in tears. Every now and then she would get close to Toñito and kiss his forehead, but he pretended to be asleep. All Toñito wanted was for his mom to smile and to be drinking hot chocolate at the ranch like before.

The next day, Toñito packed the little he had and sadly got ready to leave this destination filled with happiness and fun behind. And like my grandma used to say, the sweetness of the gum has disappeared.

New destination: Los Angeles, California.

The trip was long and confusing. Because they couldn't speak English, they almost missed their bus. Toñito wanted to learn English—so that he could take his mom around the world one day. He imagined walking with Mom in a giant city park full of snow, like the one in the book at the playpen.

"Your ID please?" A man in a green uniform asked them. Toñito's mom said nothing and handed over the paperwork in the yellow envelope that the people at the respite center had given to her.

"What's your name? Is he your little brother?" He asked.

Mom was nervous but was able to answer all the questions they had once they brought a translator. The holster on his waist scared her as much as it scared Toñito. They had spent nights shivering next to each other, days struggling to find food and water, and moments in which neither of them knew where to go next. Despite all of this, their love kept them strong, but now they were afraid. They had fled from armed men just to find more here. Mom held Toñito by his shoulders.

"We have to be strong, son. We're almost there," she whispered.

"Customs always checks that everyone on the bus is documented. They always do this at the border. They checked me while I was in Texas. I only had a visa then. I was so scared . . ." a woman said to her friend once the man got off the bus.

The next night, the bus stopped at the bus station. Toñito kept looking out the window hoping to see the uncle. He thought of what his mom had said: he had a beard and that he always wore brown boots and . . . but Toñito remembered uncle is no longer with us. He had forgotten.

"Let's go, son. I think that my aunt is already waiting for us. Hurry up, my son." Mom rushed him out of the bus as she gripped his hand tighter.

"How are we going to find her?" Toñito asked.

"Put on your sweater, you're going to get sick, the bus was hot . . ."

"Mom, I'm not cold."

"Don't disobey me, it's cold and I don't know what I would do if you got sick. PUT IT ON."

"Mom! No!"

"Do as I say, don't make me tell you again, we are in public, be prudent, Toñito. Put it on."

"¡ANTONIO!" They both turned towards the voice that shouted his name.

"You must be Antonio," a woman said.

"Oh, aunt Rosa forgive us, look I'm sorry, thank you for everything, I appreciate it very much."

"Let's go, girl," The lady cut her off.

Rosa's stare was cold, and she kept her hands in the pockets of her jacket. Toñito saw her black hair dangling on her back covering a scar on the back of her neck. She walked fast. She didn't talk or even look at us. She kept ignoring his mother's attempts to thank her, which both frustrated and worried Toñito.

"Antonio, now. Put it on," she told me again as she spread her arms to put my jacket over my shoulders.

"No, you put it on."

Slap!

Rosa's handprint on Toñito's cheek stung. Rosa kept talking but all Toñito could hear was his mother's fingers on her rosary as she prayed. Toñito could hear his mom's heartbeat and she could feel his tears over her sweater.

What if she kidnaps us? What if she hurts my mom? And if she gets rid of us because she doesn't want us? What if we have to live on the streets because she throws us out? Why does this have to happen to us? I only want for mom to not cry so much and that no one hurts us anymore, but we come to the same thing here. I don't want to be here anymore—

"Son, Son, SON, let's go!" Mom shook Toñito by the shoulder. "Ay Toñito, you're drenched in sweat, let's hope you don't catch a cold," she whispered.

Toñito wanted to tell her that he was scared. He wanted to tell her that his legs were still shaking and that he could hear his own heart jumping. He wanted to tell her that he wished we were back on the ranch with grandma. He wanted to tell her that he wanted to be eating cheese filled pupusas[4] with the family. That he wanted to go back in time like Superman to when she would tuck him in bed with a prayer and a kiss on the forehead. He wanted to say all these things to her, but he kept silent.

Toñito started having nightmares, but one kept going on through daytime. Mom would wake up every morning at 4 AM to cook Rosa's lunch for work. She would then wash and dry everyone's clothes. After lunch and before 1 o'clock, she was back to cleaning. She would grab the broom and mop and clean the entire house. Even though she was always in a rush, she usually finished just in time to cook something for Rosa. If by 6 PM dinner was not ready, Rosa would get angry. By 7 PM, she had to clean and wash dishes again and start getting ready for the next day. She had Toñito saying the good night prayer every time. Sometimes she would fall asleep from exhaustion before Toñito was done praying.

The best days were Sundays. Rosa didn't wake up until noon, so they would wake up when the sky was still dark and walk to church to hear the earliest mass. It was the only hour of the week when Toñito saw Mom at peace. They listened to the priest and sang all of the songs. They didn't have any money for the collection, but mom always said that God would understand. After church, they would take a walk to a nearby park. She would push Toñito on the swings and let him run around and play. Around 11, they would make their way back to Rosa's house. Toñito was always sad on the way back.

Toñito wanted to know why his mom sometimes had bruises on her arms. They were small and less frequent at first, but now they were a lot bigger, and colorful. Mom would say that she'd get them from when she'd trip while cleaning.

Toñito wanted to know why he couldn't join the rest of the children on the yellow bus every weekday.

"One day, when you're older, I'll explain, son," she would always say.

On the days that Toñito was really bored, he began to stare out the window. He would count the cars that would go by and watch the other children playing outside. The boy next door would get home in the yellow bus and an hour later he would come out with a soccer ball.

The first time that he saw Toñito looking at him through the window, Toñito pulled the curtains and ran away. The next day when he went outside to play, Toñito peeked through a small open sliver in the curtains. The boy kept looking at the window.

A couple of days passed before Toñito got bored enough to open the curtain again. The boy waved. He waved back. Toñito wasn't allowed to go outside, but he really wanted to go play with the ball. He had a ball just like that one in El Salvador.

Mom was still out doing the laundry. She wouldn't be back for another hour. If Toñito went outside now, mom wouldn't notice, so he ran out the door.

"Hi, my name is Toñito. Can I play soccer with you?" He asked the boy.

"Hi, Toñito. I'm Marcos. I don't have a football, but we can play with my soccer ball," he replied.

Toñito didn't understand what he said. He spoke fast, but he said soccer. So he moved his feet, and he stole the ball that was secured under his foot.

"Hey, come back!" He yelled. He started running after Toñito.

Toñito made it close to the trashcans and kicked and aimed the ball between them. When the ball went through, he jumped and screamed: "¡GOOOAL!" It had been a long time since he had played soccer. I had forgotten the emotion of the sport and how fun it was.

"That was an awesome shot!" Marcos said as he high fived Toñito. The boys took turns taking shots at the trashcans, being goalies, and kicking the ball to each other. They had so much fun, but Toñito needed to get back inside soon before his mom got home.

"One more," Toñito raised one finger. "Then I need to go home." He pointed at the house. Marcos nodded and began running toward the trashcans where Toñito was holding guard. After the game was over, Toñito ran home just before my mom got there.

Marcos's friendship made the days go by faster and life a lot sweeter. It was all going well until that day.

Marcos got near and kicked the ball. He tried to grab the ball in midair, but it hit Toñito straight in the face.

"Ahh!" Toñito screamed, with a burning sensation on his face.

Marcos ran toward him. "Are you okay? I'm so sorry. I didn't mean to hit your head. Can you stand up?"

My head hurts so much. I can't get up. I feel dizzy. He saw Marcos run away. "Where are you going?" He tried to yell, but it came out like a soft whisper.

Toñito tried to get up, but he felt disoriented and lost. It hurt so much. He couldn't open his eyes. He heard footsteps. "Are you okay?" A soft, melodic voice asked.

Toñito couldn't reply. "Mom, he doesn't speak English," said Marcos.

Toñito worried about what his mom would think, he knew she would be upset.

"Marcos, please grab another chair for Toñito's mom," Toñito opened his eyes slowly, feeling pressure and pain in his head. Toñito couldn't get up. He felt nauseous.

"Toñito is going to be . . . he's going to be okay, Miss. Please have a seat. Would you like a coffee?"

"Are you sure he's going to be okay? What happened to him? I always leave him inside. I always tell him to not go outside because something could happen to him and we don't know anybody." Her voice trailed off.

"Yes, he's going to be okay. Marcos told me he kicked the soccer ball and accidentally hit Toñito in the head. I'm a nurse. If he feels bad, we can take him to the doctor." There was her melodic voice.

"I don't have money for a doctor," his mom said softly.

"Don't worry. What's your name?"

"Marta and you?"

"My name is Hope, or in Spanish, Esperanza."

"What a beautiful name."

"Thank you, Marta. Look, your son will be fine. It was nothing more than a hit. Nothing happened to him, and he will be fine here," Hope reassured her. "Are you going to want a coffee?"

"Yes, thank you very much."

"Well. Let me get you the coffee . . . where are you from? Your accent sounds different," said Hope as she whipped up a coffee.

"We are from El Salvador."

"Wow, how far. Is it pretty there? My parents are from Colombia."

"My country is beautiful, but the violence has ruined it. There is too much violence and a comfortable life is impossible. We had been living in the shadows for a couple of years already because of all the gangs around us."

"How scary . . . what a fright. Is that why you are here in the United States?" She asked amidst the clinking sound of the coffee cups being set on the table.

"We're here for lots of reasons," his mom said slowly sipping her coffee.

"That's ok. How do you like the U.S.? There are many very nice places here."

"We don't have much money. I clean and cook for my uncle's wife. We don't have much time to go out."

"And do you get paid for cleaning the house?"

"Mmm no, but I'm very grateful to my aunt. And it's the only thing she asks for letting us stay in her house for free."

"And do you have another job?" she asked.

"Right now, I don't have a job. I don't speak English and well I don't have time with my aunt's housework. And I also don't want to leave Toñito alone for very long."

"Oh, I understand you. I also don't like to leave Marcos alone. And now that I'm separated from my husband, it is harder for me to work the night shift."

"You leave the kid alone at night?"

"No, I leave him here at my mother's house, but my mom is getting old and I don't like to leave both of them alone."

Toñito started to feel a little better. He sat up. "Mom?" he croaked.

"Oh Toñito, how are you feeling? Does your head hurt a lot? I had such a scare, son." Mom ran toward him.

"My head hurts a lot but I'm feeling a little better already."

"Miss Hope, thank you so much for all of your help. I don't know how I will be able repay you. Toñito and I need to go back to my aunt's house now."

"Don't worry about it, Marta. The doors of my house and my mother's house will always be open for you two."

"Thank you, Hope."

They trudged their way back to Tia Rosa's house dreading what awaited them.

"Where have you been, stupid girl? Ungrateful! I don't ask you for much considering all I do for you and your little son. I had no reason to accept you into my home. I don't even know you!" Rosa yelled at Marta and smacked her cheek, which resonated louder than her voice.

"Miss Marta, what's going on?!" Hope and Marcos stood outside watching Rosa.

"What's going on is this spoiled little girl didn't have dinner ready for me when I got home. Who knows where this disgraceful skank was or better yet who she was with? Right? Whore."

Slap! Rosa's hand landed on Marta's face again.

Suddenly, Hope was at my mother's side. "Ma'am! You have no right to hit this woman! She was with me. Her son wasn't well and I was taking care of him."

"Oh yeah? Okay, well then, this girl and her son are no longer my problem. Get your things and get out my sight."

Marta sobbed uncontrollably shouting in between breaths, "Oh my God!" And sighing saying, "What are we going to do now?"

"Marta and Toñito are coming with me."

"Let's go son, come on," Marta said to him amidst tears.

When Toñito woke up, Marta told him to go to the car. He saw Marcos throw bags of snacks and waters into the backseat of the car. Hope was in the driver's seat. He held his mother's hand tight.

"Tony?" Hope called out. No one had ever called Toñito by that name, but he liked it. "Don't worry, everything will be fine."

Sometimes family is who you want them to be and not who happens to be.

"Here, it's going to get cold." Hope took her jacket and gave it to his mom.

"No, I'm okay," Marta replied in a broken voice.

"You have to be strong for you and Tony." Hope kept trying to calm them down.

"We won't leave you alone; come on, Marcos!" said Hope with a smile.

The drive was beautiful. Toñito cleaned the tears from his mom's face and kissed her forehead. She prayed next to him, and Toñito felt her warmth cover his face as he fell asleep on her.

"Son, It's here. We have arrived," Mom whispered to him.

There was no sun in the sky but there were lights all over the small yet pretty house. Christmas lights. The moment Toñito got out the car he felt a cool breeze on his face. Marta came from behind screaming . . .

"Son, we're free!"

"Welcome!" Hope screamed with joy.

"I forgot to give you this," Marcos handed Toñito a backpack with one, diagonal strap. "You're going to need it when you go to school with me."

"You're going to go to school with Marcos, Tony," said Hope.

"I'm going to school with you?" Toñito jumped with excitement. "Mom, mom! Am I going to go to school with Marcos?"

Mom smiled at him.

"Yes Toñito, you'll go to school with Marcos. We can register you next week. But now we have a lot to do. Now, who is hungry?" Hope asked. Everyone said I am. Everyone ran inside the blue house, their new home. At the door, there was sign that read, "dream."

From that day on, they lived in a home and not just in a house. Having Hope and Marcos with them was always joyful and safe. Marta took care of

Marcos at night when Hope had the night shift at the hospital. Hope also got Toñito's mom a cleaning job at the hospital and she was able to make a good living for them. From that day on, Toñito no longer saw bruises on her. And other than for the times she would cut onions for the soup, she no longer cried. The years in school flew by. After a couple of months in a creative writing club in high school, Toñito began writing stories for competitions and even got to travel to other places to compete with other children from schools from all over the country.

In college, Toñito decided to pursue writing. He found solace in writing. Although there was misery and sadness in his journey to the United States, the bliss of seeing his mother so proud of him walking across the stage on his graduation day was worth it.

They still saw Marcos and Hope on occasions. Hope was offered a better job in San Francisco. It was an offer she couldn't refuse. They kept in contact and made sure to reunite at least once a year.

Toñito and his mother were granted Refugee status, which allowed them to stay in the United States. It was a difficult process; both legally and emotionally. His mom explained what physical assault and rape meant and how she had been a victim of both many times. His mom also had to explain that they had been threatened in El Salvador. If they went back, they were sure to meet their deaths. That day Toñito sat next to her in silence, listening to the sound of her heart. Eventually, they were granted Legal Permanent Resident status. They celebrated that day, cherishing the opportunity to stay in this country. There's a beautiful, joyful glint in his mother's eyes. Together, they smile at their found destination.

Notes

1. Looking for Destiny/Destination.
2. Destiny or destination.
3. *Destino* translates to destiny or destination. Throughout this text, italics are used to reflect when Spanish was utilized in the original text.
4. Pupusa: traditional Salvadorian dish of a thick corn tortilla stuffed with a filling.

· 5 ·

YESSICA COLIN

While conducting research at a school in Texas that admitted and helped immigrants, Colin listened to Camila's story. Being an immigrant herself, Colin readily understood what it is like to be a young woman who seeks to provide for herself and her family. Nicaraguan Camila decided to determine her own fate and embarking in a journey full of uncertainty, nostalgia, and strength.

Camila

Camila was destined to misery, or at least so she thought. A sudden burst into her room interrupted the million thoughts whirling around her head. It was Rafa, Charly's friend from the neighborhood. With a distraught face he said,

"Camila, Charly fell from his bike and is bleeding bad!" Alarmed, Camila quickly wiped her tears and ran along with Rafa to help Charly.

"Ouch!" said Charly in pain as his sister wiped the blood from his left hand once they were inside the house.

"It'll be ok," Camila assured her brother.

"At least you didn't smash into Mrs. Lupita's stand," laughed Rafa. Mrs. Lupita ran an *aguas frescas* stand on the corner—down the street from where Charly and Camila lived.

"Yeah, to avoid crashing into her stand I landed in a pothole and flew into rocks and now I am paying for it!" blurted Charly, upset.

"I better get going. I'll see you around, Charly" said Rafa. Both Camila and Charly waved goodbye and were left in silence. It was a hot humid day. The sun was beginning to fade, but the birds chirped and sang as if it was broad daylight. Without saying a thing, Camila leaned over the mini fridge and grabbed a mango. She sliced the mango from both sides and offered half to Charly.

Charly gulped the juicy mango and asked, "Where's grandma?" Reminded of her situation, Camila tried to hide her sad expression. How could she tell Charly about their grandma? Their grandma's health had been deteriorating rapidly and Camila did not know how to handle and cope with everything all at once. Sara, Camila's grandma, was suffering from Alzheimer's, a degenerative disease that destroys memory and other mental functions. Camila's grandma was often found wandering around completely lost by local neighbors. Some days her memory seemed ok, while other days it seemed she did not even recognize herself. The symptoms were clear and confirmed by doctors.

"She went to the market with Mrs. Lupita," replied Camila.

"It seems like every day she is getting worse," said Charly, observing his sister's face closely.

"She will get better," assured Camila, hiding her hopelessness. Charly left the kitchen table and went to rest on the couch. Camila could not stop thinking about their grandma. Everything changed and seemed to go downhill after their father's death.

Rogelio, Camila's father, stole money from a gang leader and this decision cost him his life. Camila, now in her room, cried silently, remembering her father's death. She remembered how her grandmother uncapped her father's bottle of whisky just days after his death and how she drank and cried. They had tried to adapt and adjust to their new life, but it wasn't easy. Camila had learned to care for herself and for Charly.

The next day Camila decided to visit her aunt, Margarita who lived some houses down the street. Margarita had taken care of her and Charly on numerous occasions. Camila did not know who else to rely on.

"Good morning *tía*," said Camila shyly.

"Camila, come on in. What brings you around?" asked Margarita warmly.

"Everything" said Camila. "Grandma is only getting worse. Even when she talks, she doesn't make sense. I want to go to the other side, but Charly worries me."

"To the United States?" asked Margarita, surprised. "Oh Camila, don't you know it is very hard to make it across safely? Smugglers are getting more expensive each day and only steal from the good people. It's very dangerous Camila."

"I know *tía*. I need to earn money to get my grandma some help." Margarita looked at Camila and a worried expression covered her face. She knew Camila had gone to her house to ask her to watch over Charly. "How are you going to do it, Camila?"

"I have a friend. Do you remember Melissa? Well, she is leaving on Wednesday and her uncle is a smuggler and is crossing her for free. Maybe she can get me a spot if I give her uncle my savings."

"My goodness!" exclaimed Margarita.

"If you can just please take care of Charly for the time that I will be gone. I promise—as soon as I make it across—I will find work and send you everything I have."

"Camila," Margarita said, "you do know your brother will be very sad if you leave?"

Camila started crying. She knew Charly would feel abandoned, but this was the only way to better their lives. Margarita consoled Camila and gave her an old rag to wipe her eyes.

"I will take care of Charly and will watch after your grandma. After all, we are family," Margarita said.

"I am going to talk to Charly and grandma. I will let them know my plans and tell them I will be gone for just some time, until I come back," Camila said.

Later that day, as Camila was gathering her things, she thought of how she was going to talk to Charly about her trip to the United States. She was already heartbroken at the thought of leaving her brother all by himself. She decided to write a letter:

Charly, my little brother, I am leaving to the United States for some time and will be back very soon. I am leaving to earn money to help grandma and her condition. I have already spoken to our aunt, and she will be here by the time you get home from school. She will look after you and grandma. I will be sending money very soon and our aunt will buy you everything you need. I will call you very soon. Please understand the situation and take care of grandma for me. Don't let her forget who we are. I promise I'll be back. I know you'll understand. I'll be safe; I promise

I'll take care of myself and I want you to do the same. I love you my little brother,
Camila.

By the time she finished writing, a pool of tears had wet her soft pink shirt. She folded the note and left it on the wooden table in her bedroom. She would hide it there until it was time to leave.

When that day arrived, Camila felt more anxious than she had expected. She had already gathered her most essential things and she put them in a backpack. Among them was a picture of her grandma feeding Charly some yogurt when he was younger. Camila hoped this picture would give her strength. She walked over to her bed and leaned down to reach for her piggy bank. As she lifted it in her arms, above her head, she began crying. She felt scared and wanted to run to her grandma, but she knew her grandma wouldn't understand.

It was around noon when Camila walked out of the only place she had ever known. Charly would be coming home soon to the note she had put on their kitchen counter, and it would break his heart. There was no turning back. Camila headed to the coin changer to exchange all her coins into *córdobas*. Her savings, 6,300 *córdobas*, were close to 200 U.S. dollars. Melissa's uncle, Marco, had agreed to cross her and Melissa had said to meet at the corner store, two blocks from her house. There, all three would leave on the bus to the city nearest to the border between Nicaragua and Honduras.

Camila had never been out of Managua. The city of Ocotal was quite busy, but it wasn't very large. The ride there was approximately 3 hours and very bumpy. Marco checked them in to an old motel and soon they were settled inside a small room with two beds. The amenities of the room were quite dusty as if nobody ever used them, but the two paintings on top of each bed gave the room a pleasant quality that didn't quite fit how Camila was feeling. Marco stepped out to use the payphone located outside to contact other people that would be crossing with them.

"Are you nervous?" asked Melissa.

"Who wouldn't be Meli? Don't tell me you aren't," asked Camila.

"I am, but I'm also excited for what awaits us," she replied.

"I really don't want us to get sent back," admitted Camila.

"We won't get sent back" Melissa interrupted. "My uncle is only taking family members and people he can trust to the North," assured Melissa. "This is not the typical border crossing where strangers tag along. Trust me, we've just got to do everything my uncle says," said Melissa reassuringly.

And, at that last statement, Camila began thinking about Marco. He was around 67 inches tall. He was of dark complexion with full wavy hair and dark brown eyes. She remembered what her own grandmother had said on one occasion "you can't trust no man, nobody, Camila." But she had to trust Marco; she had no other choice. Interrupting those thoughts, Marco came in with a man and a woman. They shyly introduced themselves, Tony and Jimena. Each carried a backpack. After some small talk, Marco announced that the group would wait in the small motel room for two others, Pedro and Lucia, who would be coming along.

The next day everyone had breakfast at the small stand across the street from the motel. The day was cloudy, but humid. Camila asked Marco if she could make a phone call. Upon his nod, she dialed her aunt's phone number using the nearest payphone.

"Hello," Margarita answered.

"Tía! It's me, Camila. I was just calling to see how everything is going," she said, afraid of her response.

"Hi Camila. What can I say? Charly is very sad. He didn't want to eat anything yesterday or this morning. He'll be okay but you will need to talk to him soon," advised Margarita. "Grandma is alright," she went on to say.

"I will talk to them," whispered Camila. "I will once I'm in the States, which according to Melissa's uncle should be in about a week and a half. I don't want to worry them meanwhile."

"Don't forget, Camila," said Margarita, reminding and warning her of her duty.

She knew her aunt was just trying to help and appreciated it, even if it stung. Camila walked back to the group to find two new travelers had arrived. Pedro was tall and very thin, while Lucia was short and petite. Both seemed of good nature. They exchanged introductions and all continued eating.

Per the CA4-Treaty or the Central America-4 Border Control Agreement, the Central American nations of El Salvador, Guatemala, Honduras, and Nicaragua allow their citizens to travel freely across borders. This meant the group could travel safely by bus without having to undergo any checkpoints. By the time they were on the way to Tecún-Umán, the Guatemalan city nearest the Mexican border, Camila had seen three different countries: Guatemala, El Salvador, and Honduras.

By the time they reached the bus terminal of Tecun-Uman, Camila was exhausted. After getting off the bus, everyone, including Marco, took the time to make phone calls. Camila phoned home, but nobody answered. They had probably gone to the market. Her heart was up to her throat and Camila wanted to burst out crying, but she knew she had to be strong.

The group went to the bank of the Suchiate River, a river that divides Mexico and Guatemala. The river, Marco had assured them, could be crossed easily, since few authorities patrolled the area. There were many guides taking people, including kids, across the river. Soon Camila was sitting on top of an improvised raft and being transported to the Mexican side of the river— Chiapas. Everything was happening so quickly and Camila, just like everyone else crossing the Suchiate River, was scared.

After crossing, the group stopped in a respite center where immigrants were given shelter to plan for their next moves in their journey to the U.S. Camila asked for the next location. "I think my uncle will get us across the border fairly easy, but it all depends on the Mexican officers. Some are harsh and cruel, while others just want money," Melissa said confidently. Marco rested on an old wooden chair and seemed to be lost in thought.

Camila noticed him; however, she did not know that Marco was scared. He had checked in with two other smugglers and both had said Mexican authorities had detained them, flooding them with questions. Marco knew he had to offer a good quantity to bribe the officers if he and his group were stopped. A clock that sat on top of a dusty TV marked a quarter after 5pm. Marco knew it was no longer safe to travel because gangs roamed after sunset. But he still wanted to give it a try before having to take even higher-risk routes.

"Tomorrow," said Marco suddenly, "we will leave early in the morning to arrive to Puerto Madero, Mexico. Mexican officers usually switch shifts between 6 and 7am and since it will be a Saturday morning, many of them will be tired and not as alert. I'm hoping we can cross while they are switching shifts. It's either that or jumping on a train." Upon hearing the word train Melissa exclaimed, "Train!? You'd said we wouldn't have to do that. You know it's dangerous and we probably wouldn't all make it," she said, lowering her head. While the rest listened, Marco replied, "Yes, it's either crossing through Puerto Madero, crossing straight to Chiapas and getting detained, or jumping on the train. I don't know about you, but it seems like we only have one option." Camila wanted to cry and began questioning the whole trip to the United States. "Was it worth it? What if I get raped? Break my ankle? Get left behind? What would happen to Charly if I died? Grandma?" These were all questions that flooded her mind.

"With luck," said Marcos, "we'll get across with no problem."

Unaware of the doubts his sister was having, Charly stood beside his grandma who was helping his aunt make fish soup. He decided to go outside where the sun was just beginning to fall. He noticed some food vendors leaving while others arrived. He was sorry his sister felt responsible for him and their grandma. He wanted to hug her. Tears began rolling, dampening the dry dirt his old shoes stepped on. He was grateful that his aunt was here with them. At least he knew that as long she was here with them; they would be ok. He just hoped Camila would also be ok. Charly went inside the house and stood close to the phone, hoping his sister would call soon.

It was exactly 6am when the group stepped out of the respite center. Marco hated the idea of traveling through the dangerous night hours, but they had no other choice if they wanted to reach Puerto Madero on time and avoid Mexican officials.

"Don't look at anybody, and be aware of your surroundings," warned Marco. "Gang members are always looking for easy targets that look afraid. Just act like you belong," he continued as the group walked to a combi, a bus that would transport them to their desired location.

"Marco," said Camila quickly, "what if there are Mexican officers? What do we do?"

"We all retreat with caution," he said. Camila and Melissa, Tony and Jimena, Pedro and Lucia all walked in pairs, pretending to only know one another and not the rest of the group. Marco walked in front of everyone and would signal to the rest. Camila walked alongside Melissa and accidentally made eye contact with a man who wore a blue and white striped shirt. He had wrinkles and skin burnt from the sun. Maybe he was a fisherman, or an undercover officer. Camila looked away immediately but feared that her mistake could cost the whole group's effort to make it to the land of opportunities. "Damn it, Camila. Just look ahead. How hard is that?" She thought. Marco signaled the group, and a wave of relief filled their entire bodies. Fooling the surveillance of the migration agents, each pair sped up, but as Melissa and Camila were about to cross a man yelled, "Excuse me! Ma'am!"

"Oh no!" Camila and Melissa thought.

"Damn it!" said Marco, who observed from behind a small building along with the rest of the group.

"Who's that man?" asked Jimena, worried.

Camila and Melissa slowly turned fearing the worst when the man in the blue and white striped shirt handed Camila a handkerchief she had accidentally dropped.

"Here you go young lady," he said kindly. "I thought you would need it."

"Thank you," said Camila shyly hoping he was unable to hear her loud heartbeat.

"Thank you!" exclaimed Melissa, relieved he wasn't an officer. She gently pulled Camila back to crossing the port and stared into her eyes, assuring her they were safe.

"What the hell was that?" Marco whispered loudly as they met him.

"He handed Camila a handkerchief she had dropped," Melissa replied. The whole group exhaled with relief and joy. Even Marco, who always seemed serious, cheered at their small victory.

"Unbelievable," he said, smiling.

Camila was still agitated by the thought of being detained and sent back after everything she had gone through. There was no turning back. "We are closer than ever, guys. We've got to give it all or we risk being sent home," she said out loud realizing she had just shared what was supposed to be a private thought. Everyone nodded and continued walking behind Marco.

Marco checked in at a motel in Chiapas with Camila and Melissa. Tony and Jimena and Pedro and Lucia would each check in separately to avoid any suspicion. It was more money, but the safest way to do it. After eating breakfast, everyone rested in their rooms. Meanwhile, Marco talked on his cell phone to the other smugglers. The plan was to travel by bus all the way to Tamaulipas where they would cross Matamoros and Reynosa to enter the United States. That's the route Marco knew the best and it was known to be safer than Tijuana. The bus ride to Tamaulipas would take about 2 days with stops to rest and refuel. Then they would settle in a migrant house where Lao, a smuggler and Marco's friend, was waiting. A migrant house was a house owned by one of the smugglers where immigrants being transported were allowed to wait until it was safe to cross. Of course, they all chipped in with some money; nothing here was free or given out of kindness. Marco did not know how long they would have to wait there. It was all a matter of the time, day, gangs, and bribes; these things would determine when they could cross to the United States. Camila thought about calling Charly, but before she could, she fell asleep sitting down on the bed.

When she woke up, blankets covered her body and faint sunrays were peeking through the small window shining on her face. Who knew she would now be in Mexico when just a couple of days ago she had never left her native Managua? Next to her laid Melissa, snoring softly. Her light brown hair covered most of her face, except her flecked nose. Camila reminisced about their friendship. Unlike her, Melissa lived with both of her parents. Melissa's mother was sweet and cozy, while her father was a gambler. His gambling brought Melissa's family many troubles, but they always managed to stay together. Now her parents wanted her to achieve the American dream since her opportunities in Nicaragua were limited. The distant rumbles of big trucks on the highway shook Camila away from her thoughts. They had to get going. By the time Marco entered the room, everyone was ready to go. Camila decided to call her aunt Margarita once they reached Tamaulipas.

Filled with worry, Charly was waiting for her sister's call. Why hadn't Camila called? What if she forgot about him, or even worse, what if something bad happened to her? What Charly didn't know was that his sister was the closest either of them had ever been to reaching a land that would grant them new opportunities.

When the group reached Tamaulipas, Camila found herself in a migrant house where another fifteen people were also waiting to cross. There was a grandmother with a young child and another grandmother with a newborn. She realized everyone had fled from their home countries in search of a better life; they fled for necessity, not by choice. Staying in their countries meant dying. The plan was in place: Camila and Melissa would cross with Marco; two other people would come along with them. They would ride in a car and use borrowed passports. Most of the time, the authorities just quickly glanced at the passport picture and the supposed visitor. If the person didn't seem nervous or suspicious and answered everything without any errors, they were welcomed into the United States. Camila was given little time to practice her lines, but she memorized everything verbatim. Marco also made sure everyone looked decent and not like they had just crossed through three countries. He had gone to a local Walmart where he bought some clothing and personal belongings. Camila wore a blue blouse and black pants.

As they waited for their turn to reach the U.S. checkpoint, officers walked alongside cars with dogs. When it was their turn to pull forward, a tall and slender officer greeted them. Camila had never really seen a *gringo* that close before.

"Where are you headed, Sir?" he asked, and Marco cheerfully replied, "San Antonio, Texas."

"Reason of visit?" the officer asked.

"Vacation," Marco said.

"May I see everyone's passports please?"

Camila was hot. Suddenly, she thought of her family.

"First and last name?" the officer finally asked Camila after questioning everyone else.

"Yvette Mondragon" she replied. He stared at the passport and Camila stared at everything in her field of vision except the officer's eyes. She could not control the racing thoughts in her head: "Was he going to ask her to step out of the car? Was he able to notice the slight differences between her and the picture? Had this journey come to an end?"

"Everything seems in order," the officer said handing Camila the passport back. "Drive ahead and follow that second line of cars," he instructed Marco with his hand. "Welcome to the United States." There was silence in the car. They had made it and even though everyone wanted to scream with joy, they pretended like they were really going on vacation.

"Hello? *Tía*? Grandma? Can you hear me? Is anybody there?" Camila kept saying as she was bursting with excitement. The drive to San Antonio was long and Camila had fallen asleep for most of the ride. Finally, they reached a motel. From there, Camila eagerly phoned home.

"Camila?" Charly spoke softly. He had missed his sister and hearing her voice felt as if a heavy rock was lifted of his chest.

"Charly?!" Camila exclaimed in disbelief. Tears came out of her eyes without any resistance.

"I made it, Charly," she said, feeling the great distance between them.

"You had me worried. I thought something had happened—"

"No, Charly. I'm great! And everything will be better from now on," Camila said as she cleaned her tears of joy.

Two weeks had passed, and Camila sat on her twin bed contemplating the quiet morning that surrounded her. She shared a room with Melissa in a house where the two of them lived with Marco. Camila had found a job at the Chicken Buffet across the street and was paid minimum wage, which seemed like a lot to her. Camila thought the streets were very wide and was surprised at the fact that not many people walked. Back in Nicaragua, streets were narrow, and everyone walked or biked. Every day, as she walked to work, she looked intently at people sitting in traffic in their cars. People looked different. To her surprise a lot of people also spoke Spanish. When payday finally arrived, Camila was excited to send money back home and gave her aunt specific instructions to buy Charly the best shoes she could find from *Don Antonio's Zapateria*. She also sent some money for the family's expenses and necessities. The rest was to pay her share of rent and buy groceries.

Camila was going to attempt to enroll in *Alamo High School* she looked around and liked the school. It was small and made her feel comfortable.

"Hello, I'm Alicia. Welcome! Do you need help?" a young secretary asked.

"*¿Español?*" Camila asked shyly.

"Yes! How can I help you Miss. . . ." she said, switching to Spanish.

"Camila!" Camila exclaimed and giggled in relief upon hearing her native language. "I would like to join this school, but I don't know the process. I recently moved here from Nicaragua, and I want to continue my education," Camila said, hoping her legal status wouldn't be an issue.

"Of course! I can explain how everything works!" said Alicia with a wide smile. Camila did not know if school was going to be difficult. She was afraid her lack of schooling—for years now—would be a problem. Alicia was nice, but what about the rest? Camila tried to stop doubting, knowing she needed to take advantage of all the opportunities this new country offered.

On the first day Camila arrived at the school, she pretended to be confident; nobody would want to get to know her if she seemed timid. Alicia was at the front desk when Camila entered the office and warmly greeted her and handed her the schedule. Just as Alicia began explaining where her classes would be located, a middle-aged woman with frizzy blonde hair interrupted Alicia.

"Pardon me," she said to Camila. As the woman whispered to Alicia, Camila felt a bit intimidated and overwhelmed mainly for the language barrier she faced.

"Mrs. Clay, this is Camila and she just arrived from Nicaragua and I was just telling her where her classes are located. She has English with you!"

"Oh great! Camila, it is nice to meet you. I am Mrs. Clay, your English teacher," she said in Spanish.

"Very nice to meet you, Mrs. Clay. I will try my hardest to learn English!" Camila said enthusiastically. Mrs. Clay chuckled and offered to show Camila around.

"What part of Nicaragua are you from, Camila?"

"Managua" she replied.

"My best friend from high school was from there too. Do you have any siblings that will be coming to this school too?" Mrs. Clay asked slowly trying to use perfect Spanish.

"No, my only sibling is Charly and he stayed back in Nicaragua. He's only twelve."

"Oh, I see . . ." Mrs. Clay said intrigued.

Camila entered her first class, art, and saw some people already seated. She had nothing but a small binder with scratch paper and a pencil. As Mrs. Lopez, the art teacher, handed out some sketch pencils she welcomed Camila and handed her a sheet of expectations for the class. She was glad she was now attending a better school in the United States.

At lunch, Camila was amazed that free food was given. If she had known this, she wouldn't have made herself a bean sandwich and potatoes in the morning. Extra food was never a problem, however. The cafeteria was big, and everyone seemed to have friends. As Camila picked up her food tray, she also grabbed some cookies and chips. The vendor staring at Camila waited for her to hand her some money. But Camila simply smiled and tried to walk away. As the woman noticed Camila trying to dupe her, she began raising her voice telling Camila she could not take the cookies and chips without paying for them. Camila did not understand and began blushing when suddenly a girl behind her intervened. She told the vendor she would pay for it and told Camila in Spanish to wait for her as she paid for her things. Camila was embarrassed, but relieved that someone had intervened. After the girl paid, she walked with Camila and explained to her that the snacks were not free. Very kindly she offered for Camila to sit with her; of course, Camila agreed.

"My name is Diana by the way. Are you . . . new?" asked Diana.

"Yes, today is my first day," said Camila.

"Oh great! You will get used to this school very quickly. It's not that big," Diana said smiling.

"Yeah, I'm sorry that you had to pay for my food. I did not understand. I just arrived in the U.S from Nicaragua and I'm learning the way of things," Camila said.

"It was nothing. Don't worry, there's a first time for everything and I am happy to help you with anything you need," Diana said with assurance.

A month after arriving to the U.S Camila found herself gradually growing more comfortable. She struggled a bit with English, but she stayed sometimes after school with Mrs. Clay to review her grammar. For Camila, Mrs. Clay was an angel. Mrs. Clay cared about her. She regularly asked Camila if she needed anything but, Camila's response was always the same—she needed her family. Back in Nicaragua, things were ok. Camila made sure to send her aunt plenty of money so that she would continue looking after her family. Charly missed Camila just as much as she missed him, but now he had new clothes and there was always food on the table. He knew his sister worked hard to send those U.S dollars, but he wanted to be with her. Just like Camila, he wanted to leave all he had ever known and go to the United States, where his big brave sister was. One Saturday night after Camila had gotten back from work, Charly called and told her about his plans.

"No, Charly!" Camila yelled at him.

"Until you forget about me?!" There was silence. Camila's anger turned into tears, "Don't say that. I would never forget about you Charly."

"That's what you say now," he cried.

"Listen I will try to figure out how we can be together. Ok?" she said, trying to stay positive. "But please. I got lucky Charly. If it wasn't for Melissa and Marco, I would not be here. I don't want bad things to happen to you because, trust me, they can and do happen. Please promise me that you will not try anything without my consent," Camila pleaded.

"Only if you promise you will try to figure a way that we can all be together," Charly replied.

The next day Camila sat in class thinking that she could not allow Charly to come to the U.S unaccompanied. At the end of the school day Camila talked to Mrs. Clay and she promised to help. She knew a very good immigration lawyer, Mario, and together they spoke to him. Mrs. Clay accompanied Camila to the appointment they had made, and assured her Mario was a good person. Nonetheless, Camila felt unsure and scared.

Mario proposed some options. Grandma and Charly could apply for a visa to get humanitarian relief, which could take months and sometimes years. They could also come illegally and apply for relief once in the United States. All of these were risky—relief was denied all the time and the courts were backlogged so they could live years in limbo. The last option, which Camila liked most, was for both of them to apply for a tourist visa. When the tourist visa expired, they could join the many immigrants who lived with expired tourist visas in the U.S.—the lawyer didn't talk about that part, but Camila knew about it.

Camila contacted her aunt and informed her about these options. She was proud of Camila for playing such a big role and being brave. They applied for the tourist visa and awaited the day of the interviews.

Camila's family was approved for their U.S tourist visa within 3 months. Nearly 6 months had passed since Camila last saw her family. She waited in the airport arrivals area and shook with excitement. She couldn't believe how drastically her life had changed and how drastically the life of her family was about to change. Camila frantically searched the face of every arrival but did not see her family. She was growing impatient. Suddenly she saw a young boy who was holding a backpack, and two women she recognized. "*Mi familia*," she thought. "Never again will we be separated," she whispered as her eyes met theirs and tears flowed down her cheeks.

Camila
Wendy Herrera (Translator)

El destino de Camila era a la miseria, o al menos eso pensaba ella. Un repentino estallido en su habitación interrumpió los muchos pensamientos que se agolpaban en su mente. Era Rafa, el amigo de Charly. Con su rostro lleno de angustia, dijo,

"¡Camila, Charly se cayó de su bicicleta y está sangrando mucho!" Alarmada, Camila, rápidamente limpió sus lágrimas y corrió junto con Rafa para ayudar a Charly.

"¡Ay!", dijo Charly, a la misma vez que su hermana limpiaba la sangre de su mano izquierda, ya dentro de la casa.

"Todo va a estar bien", Camila le aseguró a su hermano.

"Por lo menos, no te estrellaste en el puesto de la señora Lupita", Rafa se rio. La señora Lupita, dirigía un puesto de aguas frescas en la esquina de la calle, de donde vivían Charly y Camila.

"¡Sí, para evitar chocarme en el puesto, aterricé en un bache y fue a chocar contra las rocas y ahora estoy pagando por ello!" agregó molesto Charly.

"Será mejor que me vaya. Nos vemos pronto, Charly", dijo Rafa. Camila y Charly se despidieron, y luego se quedaron en silencio. Era un día caluroso y húmedo. El solo comenzaba a desvanecerse, pero los pájaros cantaban y entonaban, como si estuvieran a plena luz del día. Sin decir nada, Camila se inclinó sobre la mini-nevera y agarró un mango. Lo cortó de ambos lados y le ofreció la mitad a Charly.

Charly se comió el jugoso mango, y le preguntó: "¿Dónde está abuelita?" Recordándose de su situación, Camila intentó ocultar su triste expresión. ¿Cómo le va a poder decir a Charly, lo de su abuela? La salud de su abuela se había deteriorado rápidamente y Camila no sabía cómo manejar y lidiar con todo esto a la vez. Sara, la abuela de Camila, sufría de Alzheimer, una enfermedad degenerativa que destruye la memoria y otras funciones mentales. A la abuela de Camila se la encontraban a veces vagando por los vecindarios, pérdida por completo. Pero otros días, su memoria parecía estar bien, mientras que otros días parecía que ni siquiera se podía reconocer a sí misma. Los síntomas eran claros y confirmados por los doctores.

"Ella fue al mercado con la señora Lupita", respondió Camila.

"Parece que cada día que pasa se está poniendo peor", dijo Charly, observando de cerca, la cara de su hermana.

"Ella se mejorará", aseguró Camila, escondiendo la desesperanza que sentía. Charly, salió de la mesa de la cocina, y se fue a descansar al sofá. Camila, no podía dejar de pensar en su abuela. Todo estaba cambiando, y parecía ir cuesta abajo, después del asesinato de su padre.

Rogelio, el padre de Camila, robó dinero a un líder de las pandillas, y esta decisión le costó la vida. Camila, ahora en su habitación, lloraba silenciosamente, recordando la muerte de su padre. Ella recordó cómo su abuela destapó la botella de güisqui de su padre, pocos días después de su muerte, cómo esta bebía y lloraba. Todos habían tratado de adaptarse y de ajustarse a su nueva vida, pero no había sido fácil. Camila había aprendido a cuidar a Charly.

Al día siguiente, Camila decidió ir a visitar a su tía Margarita. Ella vivía a unas casas más abajo de la calle. Margarita había cuidado de ella y de Charly en numerosas ocasiones. Camila no sabía en quien más confiar.

"Buenos días, tía", dijo Camila tímidamente.

"Entra, Camila. ¿Qué te trae por aquí?", preguntó Margarita amablemente.

"Todo", dijo Camila. "La abuela está empeorando. Quiero irme para el otro lado, pero me preocupa Charly".

"¿A los Estados Unidos?", preguntó sorprendida Margarita. "Oh Camila, ¿no sabes que es muy difícil hacerlo? Los coyotes cada vez están cobrando más, y, además, sólo les roban a las personas buenas. Camila es muy peligroso".

"Lo sé tía. Necesito ganar dinero para ayudar a mi abuelita". Margarita miró a Camila con una expresión de preocupación. Se dio cuenta en ese momento de que Camila había ido a su casa para pedirle que cuidara a Charly. "Camila, ¿cómo vas a hacerlo?"

"Tengo una amiga. ¿Te acuerdas de Melissa? Bueno, ella se va el miércoles, y su tío, es un coyote, y la está cruzando gratis. Tal vez pueda conseguirme un lugar, si le doy a su tío todos mis ahorros".

"¡Dios mío!", exclamó Margarita.

"Si usted por favor puede cuidar de Charly por el tiempo que esté ausente, le prometo—que tan pronto cruce—voy a buscar trabajo, y le voy a enviar todo lo que tenga".

"Camila", dijo Margarita, "¿sabes que tu hermano se va a poner muy triste si te vas?"

Camila empezó a llorar. Ella sabía que Charly se sentiría abandonado, pero esta era la única manera de mejorar sus vidas. Margarita consoló a Camila y le dio un trapo viejo para que se limpiara las lágrimas.

"Voy a hablar con Charly y con la abuela. Les haré saber sobre mis planes, y les diré que me iré por un tiempo".

Más tarde ese mismo día, Camila estaba recogiendo sus cosas y pensaba cómo iba a decirle a Charly sobre su viaje a los Estados Unidos. Estaba desconsolada al pensar que dejaría a su hermano. Decidió escribirle una carta:

Charly, hermanito mío, me voy a los Estados Unidos por algún tiempo, y volveré muy pronto. Me voy a ganar dinero para ayudar con la enfermedad de la abuela. Ya hablé con nuestra tía, y ella estará aquí cuando llegues a casa después de la escuela. Ella cuidará de ti y de abuelita. Voy a enviar dinero muy pronto y nuestra tía te comprará todo lo que necesites. Te llamaré muy pronto. Por favor, yo sé que entenderás la situación y cuida de la abuela por mí. No dejes que se olvide de quienes somos. Te prometo que volveré. Sé que lo entenderás. Estaré a salvo. Te prometo que me cuidaré y quiero que hagas lo mismo. Te quiero hermanito.

Camila

Al finalizar de escribir la carta, un charco de lágrimas había mojado la camisa de color rosa palido de Camila. Dobló la nota y la dejó en la mesa de madera de su dormitorio. La escondería allí, hasta que llegara el momento de irse a los Estados Unidos.

Cuando ese día llegó, Camila, estaba más ansiosa de lo que había pensado. Ya había reunido sus cosas, las más esenciales, y las puso en la mochila que solía llevar a la escuela. Entre las cosas, había una foto de su abuela dando yogur a Charly, cuando era más pequeño. Camila esperaba que esta foto le diera fuerza. Se sintió asustada y quería correr hacía su abuela, pero sabía que su abuela no la entendería

Era casi mediodía cuando Camila salió del único lugar que ella había conocido. Charly volvería a casa pronto y encontraría la carta que había puesto en el mostrador de la cocina, la carta que le rompería el corazón. No había marcha atrás. Camila, se dirigió al cambiador de monedas, para intercambiar todas sus monedas en córdobas. Sus ahorros, 6,300 córdobas eran casi 200 dólares americanos. El tío de Melissa, Marco, había aceptado cruzarla y Melissa le había dicho que se encontraran en la tienda de la esquina, a dos cuadras de su casa. Allí, los tres se irían en el autobús a la ciudad más cercana a la frontera entre Nicaragua y Honduras.

Camila, nunca había salido de Managua. La ciudad de Ocotal estaba llena de gente, pero no era muy grande. El trayecto era de aproximadamente tres horas y el camino estaba lleno de baches. Marco las registró en un viejo motel y pronto se instalaron en la pequeña habitación, que tenía dos camas. Las comodidades de la habitación estaban todas polvorientas, como si nadie las usara, pero, las dos pinturas en la parte superior de cada cama daban una calidad agradable que no encajaba con lo que sentía Camila. Marco salió de la habitación para usar un teléfono público que estaba situado afuera y así contactar a otras personas que querían cruzar con ellos.

"¿Estás nerviosa?", preguntó Melissa.

"¿Quién no lo estaría, Meli? No me digas que tú no", preguntó Camila.

"Yo también lo estoy, pero también estoy emocionada por lo que nos espera", respondió.

"Realmente no quiero que nos manden de vuelta", Camila admitió.

"No, no nos van a devolver", interrumpió Melissa. "Mi tío sólo está llevando familiares y personas con las que él pueda confiar en el norte", Melissa le aseguró. "Este no es el típico cruce fronterizo donde personas extrañas quieren pegarse al grupo. Créeme, sólo tenemos que hacer todo lo que mi tío dice y estaremos bien", Melissa dijo.

Y con esta última afirmación, Camila empezó a pensar en Marco. Era 67 pulgadas de alto más o menos, de tez oscura, con el pelo ondulado, y los ojos marrones oscuros. Ella recordó lo que su propia abuela le había dicho en una ocasión, "no se puede confiar en ningún hombre, en nadie, Camila". Pero en esta ocasión tenía que confiar en Marco, no tenía otra opción. Marco entró con un hombre y una mujer, interrumpiendo sus pensamientos. Se presentaron tímidamente, Tony y Jimena. Cada uno llevaba una mochila. Después de un poco de charla, Marco anunció que el grupo esperaría en la pequeña habitación del motel la llegada de otros dos, Pedro y Lucía, que vendrían pronto.

Al día siguiente, todos desayunaron en el pequeño puesto que estaba al otro lado de la calle, a unos pocos metros del motel. El día estaba nublado, pero húmedo. Camila, le preguntó a Marco si podía hacer una llamada telefónica. Después de que él asintió, ella marcó el número de teléfono de su tía, usando la cabina telefónica más cerca del motel.

"Hola", contestó Margarita.

"¡Tía! Soy yo, Camila. Solo le llamaba para saber cómo va todo", dijo, con miedo de la respuesta.

"Hola Camila. ¿Qué puedo decirte? Charly está muy triste. No quería comer nada ayer y tampoco esta mañana. Él estará bien con nosotros, pero tendrás que hablar muy pronto con él", Margarita le aconsejó. "Abuela está bien", continuó diciendo.

"Hablaré con ellos", susurró Camila. "Lo haré, una vez que esté en los Estados Unidos, que, según el tío de Melissa, voy a estar en una semana y media. No quiero preocuparlos, mientras tanto."

"Camila, no te olvides", dijo Margarita, recordándole y advirtiéndole de su deber.

Ella sabía que su tía sólo estaba tratando de ayudar, y ella lo apreciaba, incluso aunque la verdad doliera. Camila regresó al grupo y encontró los dos nuevos viajeros que ya habían llegado. Pedro, era alto y muy delgado, mientras que, Lucía era bajita y pequeña. Ambos parecían ser amables. Se presentaron y todos continuaron comiendo.

Por el Tratado CA4 o el acuerdo control fronterizo centroamericano las naciones centroamericanas de El Salvador, Guatemala, Honduras y Nicaragua, sus ciudadanos pueden viajar libremente a través de las fronteras. Esto significa, que el grupo podía viajar con seguridad en autobús sin tener que someterse a ningún puesto de control. En el momento que llegaron a Tecún-Umán, la ciudad guatemalteca que está más cerca de la frontera con México, Camila había ya visto tres países diferentes, Guatemala, el Salvador y Honduras.

Cuando llegaron a la terminal de autobuses de Tecún-Umán, Camila estaba agotada. Después de bajar del autobús, todo el mundo, incluyendo a Marco, se dedicaron a hacer algunas llamadas telefónicas. Camila telefoneó a casa, pero nadie respondió. Pensó que probablemente habían ido al mercado. Se le hacía un nudo en la garganta y quería llorar, pero sabía que tenía que ser fuerte.

El grupo llegó a la ribera del Río Suchiate, un río que divide a México y Guatemala. En el río, Marco les aseguró que podían cruzarlo fácilmente puesto que hay poca vigilancia de las autoridades de la zona. Había muchos guías que cruzaban a gente, incluso a niños. Al poco, Camila estaba sentada encima de una balsa improvisada que la transportaba al lado mexicano del río—Chiapas. Todo sucedía muy rápido y Camila, como las otras personas que cruzaban el Río Suchiate, estaban asustadas.

Después de haber cruzado, el grupo se detuvo en un centro de descanso para inmigrantes, donde las personas reciben refugio, y pueden planear los próximos movimientos del viaje a los Estados Unidos. Camila preguntó sobre la siguiente ubicación. "Creo que mi tío nos va a llevar a través de la frontera fácilmente, bueno, todo depende de los oficiales mexicanos. Algunos son despiadados y crueles, mientras que otros sólo quieren dinero", dijo Melissa con confianza. Mientras las chicas hablaban sentadas sobre el cemento frío. Marco descansaba en una vieja silla de madera y parecía estar perdido en sus pensamientos.

Camila se fijó en él; sin embargo, no supo que en el fondo Marco estaba asustado. Él ya había charlado con dos contrabandistas y ambos habían dicho que las autoridades mexicanas los habían detenido, y que les habían hecho muchas preguntas. Marco sabía que tenía que ofrecer una buena cantidad de dinero para sobornar a los oficiales si fueran detenidos. El reloj que estaba encima de la televisión polvorienta marcaba un cuarto después de las cinco de la tarde. Marco sabía que después de esta hora no era seguro viajar porque las pandillas vagaban después del atardecer. Aún así debía intentarlo antes de tener que tomar rutas de mayor riesgo.

"Mañana", dijo Marco de repente. "Nos iremos temprano, en la mañana, para llegar al Puerto Madero, México. Los oficiales mexicanos usualmente cambian de turno entre las 6 y las 7 de la mañana y como será sábado muchos de ellos estarán cansados y no estarán tan alertas. Espero que podamos cruzar mientras cambien el turno. Es eso o saltar en el tren". Al escuchar la palabra tren, Melissa exclamó: "¡¡Tren!? Dijiste que no tendríamos que hacer eso. Usted sabe que es peligroso, y probablemente, no todos sobrevivirían", dijo, bajando la cabeza. Mientras el resto del grupo escuchaba, Marco respondió: "Sí, atravesamos por el Puerto Madero, cruzando directamente a Chiapas y ser detenidos, o saltar en el tren. No sé que dicen ustedes, pero parece que sólo tenemos una opción", Camila quería llorar y empezó a cuestionar todo el viaje a los Estados Unidos. "¿valdrá la pena? ¿y si me violan? ¿me romperé el tobillo? ¿me quedaré atrás? ¿Qué le va a pasar a Charly si muero? ¿abuela?", estas eran todas las preguntas que pasaban por su cabeza.

"Con suerte", dijo Marco, "cruzaremos sin ningún problema".

Sin tener conocimiento de las dudas de su hermana, Charly, estaba junto a su abuela y su tía que cocinaban sopa de pescado. Decidió ir afuera donde el sol empezaba a caer. Vio a algunos vendedores de comida alejándose mientras otros llegaban. Sintió lástima por su hermana, quien se sentía responsable por él y su abuela. Quería abrazarla. Las lágrimas empezaron a rodarle por las mejillas, humedeciendo el suelo que pisaban sus zapatos. Estaba agradecido con su tía por estar allí con ellos. Al menos sabía que mientras estuviera allí con ellos, estarían bien. Sólo esperaba que Camila también estuviera bien. Charly, se dirigió para adentro de la casa y se quedó muy cerca del teléfono, esperando que su hermana llamara pronto.

Eran exactamente las seis de la mañana cuando el grupo salió del centro de inmigrantes. Marco odiaba la idea de viajar a través de las peligrosas horas nocturnas, pero no tenían otra opción si estos querían llegar al Puerto Madero a tiempo y evitar a los oficiales mexicanos.

"No miren a nadie y estén alerta", advirtió Marco. "Los miembros de las pandillas siempre están buscando objetivos fáciles y asustados. Actúen como si fueran de esta área", continuó mientras el grupo caminaba a una combi, un autobús que los transportaría a su siguiente destino.

"Marco", dijo rápidamente Camila. "¿Y si hay oficiales mexicanos? ¿Qué hacemos?"

"Nos retiraremos con cautela", dijo. Camila y Melissa, Tony y Jimena, Pedro y Lucía caminaban en parejas, fingiendo que sólo se conocían unos a otros, y no al resto del grupo. Marco caminó delante de todo el mundo y señaló al resto. Camila caminó junto a Melissa y accidentalmente hizo contacto visual con un hombre que usaba una camisa de rayas azules y blancas. Tenía arrugas y la piel quemada por el sol. Tal vez era un pescador, o un oficial encubierto. Camila miró hacia otro lado inmediatamente, pero temía que su error pudiera costarle al grupo todo el esfuerzo dado para llegar a la tierra de las oportunidades. "Maldita sea, Camila. Sólo mira hacia adelante ¿Qué tan difícil es hacer eso?" Pensó. Marco hizo señales al grupo y un sentimiento de alivio llenó sus cuerpos. Engañando la vigilancia de los agentes de migración, cada par aceleró, pero cuando Melissa y Camila estaban a punto de cruzar un hombre gritó: "¡Discúlpeme! ¡Señora!"

"¡Oh no!" Camila y Melissa pensaron.

"¡Maldita sea!", dijo Marco que observaba desde detrás de un pequeño edificio junto al resto del grupo.

"¿Quién es ese hombre?", Jimena preguntó preocupada.

Camila y Melissa lentamente se voltearon, temiendo lo peor, cuando el hombre de la camisa de rayas azules y blancas le entregó a Camila un pequeño pañuelo que había perdido accidentalmente.

"Aquí está jovencita", dijo amablemente. "Pensé que lo necesitaría".

"Gracias", dijo Camila tímidamente con la esperanza de que no pudiera oír su corazón latir fuertermente.

"¡Gracias!", exclamó Melissa, aliviada porque no era un oficial. Suavemente empujo a Camila para que cruzara al puerto y la miró fijamente a los ojos asegurándole que todo estaba bien.

"¿Qué diablos fue eso?", Marco les susurró en voz alta cuando lo encontraron.

"Le entregó a Camila un pañuelo que se le había caído", respondió Melissa. Todo el grupo respiro con alivio y alegría. Incluso Marco, que siempre parecía estar serio, en ese momento, festejó la pequeña victoria.

"Increíble", dijo sonriendo.

Camila todavía estaba en estado de shock, la sola idea de haber sido detenida y envidada de regreso a su país, después de todo lo que había pasado, hacía que temblara de miedo. No había marcha atrás. "Estamos más cerca que nunca chicos. Tenemos que darlo todo o nos estaremos en riesgo de ser enviados a casa", dijo en voz alta, dándose cuenta de que acababa de compartir un pensamiento, algo que solamente debía estar en su cabeza. Todo el mundo asintió y siguió caminando detrás de Marco.

Marco se registró en un motel en Chiapas, con Camila, Melissa. Tony, Jimena, Pedro y Lucía se registraron por separado para evitar sospechas. Había que gastar más dinero, pero el método era más seguro. Después de desayunar, todos se marcharon a descansar en sus respectivas habitaciones. Mientras tanto, Marco, hablaba por el teléfono celular con otros contrabandistas. El plan era viajar en autobús todo el camino hasta Tamaulipas donde cruzarían a Matamoros y Reynosa para entrar a los Estados Unidos. Esa era la ruta que Marco conocía mejor era más segura que la de Tijuana. El viaje en autobús a Tamaulipas tomaría unos dos días, con paradas para descansar y cargar combustible. Después, se instalarían en una casa para inmigrantes, donde Lao, un contrabandista y amigo de Marco, estaría esperándolos. La casa no era un refugio sino una casa que los contrabandistas usaban para esconder a los inmigrantes y para que esperaran para ser transportados o que el cruce fuera seguro. Por supuesto, todos los contrabandistas habían aportado algo de dinero para comprarla, nada en este mundo es gratis o dado por bondad. Marco no sabía cuánto tiempo tenían que esperar allí. Todo era cuestión de tiempo, de las pandillas, y de los sobornos, estas cosas serían las que determinarían cuando podían cruzar a los Estados Unidos. Camila pensó en llamar a Charly, pero antes de que pudiera hacerlo, se quedó dormida, allí sentada en la cama.

Cuando se despertó, una manta le cubría el cuerpo y los rayos de sol que entraban a la habitación por una pequeña ventana brillaban en su cara. ¿Quién diría que ahora estaría en México, cuando hacía sólo un par de días ella nunca hubiera pensado dejar su natal Managua? Junto a ella dormía Melissa, roncaba suavemente. Su cabello castaño claro cubría la mayor parte de su rostro, excepto por la nariz pecosa. Camila pensaba en su amistad. A diferencia de ella, Melissa vivía con sus padres. La madre de Melissa era dulce y acogedora, mientras que su padre era un jugador. Su obsesión con el juego trajo muchos problemas a la familia de Melissa, pero siempre se las arreglaron para permanecer juntos. Y ahora, sus padres querían que ella lograra el sueño americano ya que había pocas oportunidades en Nicaragua. Los distantes sonidos de los camiones en la carretera trajeron a Camila a su realidad. Tenían que ponerse en marcha. Cuando Marco entró en la habitación, todos estaban listos. Camila decidió llamar a su tía Margarita una vez llegaran a Tamaulipas.

Lleno de preocupación, Charly esperaba la llamada de su hermana. "¿Por qué no llamaba Camila? ¿Qué tal si se olvidó de él?, o peor aún, ¿tal vez le pasó algo malo?", pensó. Lo que Charly no sabía era que su hermana estaba más cerca que cualquiera de ellos había estado en llegar a la tierra que les otorgaría nuevas oportunidades.

Cuando el grupo llegó a Tamaulipas, Camila se encontró con una casa de inmigrantes donde otras quince personas también estaban esperando para cruzar. En ese lugar, había una abuela con un niño pequeño y otra abuela con un recién nacido. Se dio cuenta de que todos habían huido de sus países de origen en busca de una vida mejor; huían por necesidad y no por elección. En muchos casos, quedarse en sus países significaba la muerte. El plan estaba decidido: Camila y Melissa cruzarían con Marco, otras dos personas vendrían con ellos. Viajarían en coche y utilizarían pasaportes prestados. La mayoría de las veces, las autoridades echan un vistazo rápidamente a la foto del pasaporte y al supuesto visitante. Si la persona no parece nerviosa o sospechosa y contesta todo sin errores son recibidos en los Estados Unidos. A Camila, le dieron poco tiempo para que practicara sus líneas, pero ello lo había memorizado todo textualmente. Marco también le aseguró de que todo el grupo se viera bien y no parecieran como si acababan de cruzar tres países. Había ido a un Walmart local donde había comprado algo de ropa y algunas cosas personales. Camila vestía una blusa azul y pantalones negros e incluso llevaba algunas joyas falsas. Marco le había asegurado que era un traje barato, pero, Camila pensó que se veía mejor que la mitad de la ropa en Managua.

Mientras esperaban su turno para llegar al punto de control de los Estados Unidos, los oficiales caminaban junto a los coches con perros. Cuando su turno llego para tirar hacia adelante, un oficial alto y delgado los saludó. Camila nunca había visto un gringo tan cerca.

"¿A dónde se dirige, señor?" preguntó, y Marco alegremente contesto: "San Antonio, Texas".

"¿La razón de la visita?", preguntó el oficial.

"Vacaciones", dijo Marco

"¿Puedo ver los pasaportes de todos, por favor?"

Camila sentía calor. De repente, pensó en su familia.

"¿Nombre y apellido?", el oficial finalmente le preguntó a Camila, después de interrogar a todos los demás.

"Yvette Mondragón", respondió ella. Se quedó mirando al pasaporte y Camila se quedó mirando en su campo de visión, excepto a los ojos del oficial. No podía controlar los pensamientos que pasaban por su cabeza: "¿Será que me va a pedir que salga del coche? ¿habrá notado las ligeras diferencias entre la foto y yo? ¿Será que ha llegado el fin de este viaje?"

"Todo parece estar en orden" dijo el oficial que le entregaba el pasaporte a Camila. "Avance y siga la segunda línea de coches", instruyó a Marco con la mano. "Bienvenido a los Estados Unidos". Hubo silencio en el coche. Lo habían logrado, y aunque todos querían gritar de alegría, tuvieron que fingir que realmente iban de vacaciones.

"¿Hola? ¿Tía? ¿Mamá? ¿Me escuchan? ¿Hay alguien allí?", Camila decía, mientras que estallaba de emoción. El viaje a San Antonio había sido largo y Camila se había quedado dormida durante la mayor parte del viaje. Finalmente, llegaron a un motel. Desde allí, Camila llamó ansiosamente a casa.

"¿Camila?" Charly dijo en voz baja. Había añorado a su hermana y escuchar su voz era como si le hubieran quitado una roca pesada de encima.

"¡¿Charly?!", Camila exclamó. Las lágrimas salieron de sus ojos sin parar.

"Lo hice, Charly, te he echado mucho de menos", dijo, sintiendo la gran distancia que había entre ellos.

"Me tenías preocupado. Pensé, que algo te había sucedido",

"No Charly, ¡Estoy muy bien! Y todo será mejor a partir de hoy", dijo Camila, mientras limpiaba sus lágrimas de alegría.

Ya habían pasado dos semanas y Camila estaba sentada en su cama pequeña contemplando tranquila aquella mañana. Compartía una habitación con Melissa, en una casa donde ambas vivían con Marco. Camila había encontrado un trabajo en el Chicken Buffet, al otro lado de la calle y le pagaban el salario mínimo, lo cual le parecía mucho. Como el trayecto era corto, caminaba al trabajo. Camila pensó que las calles eran muy amplias y se sorprendió que no muchas personas caminaran. En Nicaragua las calles eran estrechas y todo el mundo caminaba o andaba en bicicleta. Todos los días, de camino a su trabajo, miraba fijamente a las personas que estaban sentadas en los carros en el tráfico. Las personas se veían diferentes. Para su sorpresa, muchas personas también hablaban español. Cuando finalmente llegó el pago, Camila estaba emocionada de enviar dinero a casa, ella le dio a su tía instrucciones específicas sobre qué comprar. Para Charly, los mejores zapatos que se pudieran encontrar en la zapatería de Don Antonio. Ella también envió algo de dinero para otras necesidades de la familia. Con el resto del dinero pagó parte del alquiler y comida.

Camila iba a tratar de inscribirse en la preparatoria Álamo, miró a su alrededor y le gustó la escuela. Era pequeña y la hacía sentirse más cómoda y menos intimidada que la primera escuela.

"Hello, I'm Alicia. Welcome! Do you need help?": ("Hola, Soy Alicia. ¡Bienvenida! ¿necesitas ayuda?"), preguntó la joven secretaria.

"*¿Español?*" tímidamente Camila preguntó.

"¡Sí! ¿Cómo la puedo ayudar Srta....?", dijo, cambiando al español.

"¡Camila!" exclamó y se rio con alivio al escuchar su lengua materna. "Me gustaría inscribirme en esta escuela, pero no conozco el proceso. Hace poco me mudé de Nicaragua y quiero continuar con mi educación", dijo Camila, esperando que su estatus legal no fuera un problema.

"¡Por supuesto! ¡Yo puedo explicarle cómo funciona todo!" dijo Alicia con una gran sonrisa. Camila no sabía si la escuela iba a ser difícil. Ella temía que los años que no había asistido a la escuela la afectaran. Alicia era muy simpática, pero ¿y el resto? Camila intento dejar de dudar, ya que sabía que tenía que aprovechar todas las oportunidades que este nuevo país le ofrecía.

El primer día que Camila llegó a la escuela fingió tener confianza; nadie querría conocerla si aparentaba ser tímida. Alicia estaba en la recepción cuando Camila entró en la oficina y la saludó calurosamente y le entregó el programa escolar. Mientras Alicia le comenzaba a explicar a Camila donde se ubicaban sus clases, una mujer adulta, con cabello rubio rizado interrumpió a Alicia.

"Perdóneme" le dijo la mujer a Camila. La mujer le susurró algo a Alicia, Camila se sintió un poco intimidada y abrumada, principalmente por la barrera del idioma.

"Señora Clay, ella es Camila y acaba de llegar de Nicaragua y ahora le estaba diciendo dónde están sus clases. ¡Tiene la clase de inglés con usted!"

"¡Oh, genial! Camila, es un placer conocerte. Soy la señora Clay, su maestra de inglés", ella dijo en español.

"Es un placer conocerla señora Clay. ¡Voy a tratar de aprender inglés lo más pronto posible!" dijo muy entusiasmada Camila. La señora Clay se rio y se ofreció a mostrarle el resto de la escuela.

"¿De qué parte de Nicaragua eres Camila?"

"Managua", ella respondió.

"Mi mejor amigo de la secundaria era también de allí. ¿Tiene usted algún hermano que vaya a venir a esta escuela también?", la señora Clay le preguntó lentamente, tratando de usar el español perfectamente.

"No, mi único hermano es Charly y se quedó en Nicaragua; sólo tiene doce años".

"Oh, ya veo . . .". La señora Clay dijo algo intrigada.

Camila entró a su primera clase, la de arte, y vio algunas personas que ya estaban sentadas. No tenía nada más que una pequeña carpeta con papel y un lápiz. Mientras la señora López, la maestra de arte, le entregó algunos lápices para dibujar y le dio la bienvenida a Camila, también le entregó una hoja de expectativas para la clase. Ella se alegró, porque ahora tenía la oportunidad de asistir a una mejor escuela en los Estados Unidos.

En el almuerzo, Camila se sorprendió, porque la comida que le dieron era gratis. Si ella hubiera sabido esto, ella no se hubiera hecho un sándwich de frijol y patatas en la mañana. La comida extra no iba a ser un problema, sin embargo. La cafetería era grande, y todos parecían tener amigos. Cuando Camila recogió su bandeja de comida, también tomó algunas galletas y patatas fritas. La vendedora se quedó mirando a Camila y esperó a que le pagará. Camila simplemente sonrió y trató de alejarse. Como la mujer pensó que Camila trataba de engañarla, comenzó a levantar la voz diciéndole que no podía tomar las galletas y las patatas fritas y no pagarlas. Camila no entendió y comenzó a sonrojarse, cuando de repente, una chica intervino. Ella le dijo a la vendedora que pagaría por ella, y le dijo a Camila en español, que la espe-rara mientras pagaba por sus cosas. Camila estaba avergonzada, pero aliviada que alguien hubiera intervenido. Después de pagar, la muchacha caminó con Camila y le explicó que no todo eran gratis. Amablemente se ofreció para que Camila se sentará con ella, por supuesto que Camila aceptó.

"Por cierto, me llamo Diana ¿eres . . . nueva?", preguntó Diana

"Sí, hoy es mi primer día", dijo Camila.

"¡Oh, genial! Te acostumbrarás a esta escuela rápidamente. No es muy grande", Diana dijo sonriendo.

"Oh, siento mucho que tuvieras que haber pagado por mi comida. No entendía nada de lo que me estaba diciendo. Acabo de llegar a los Estados Unidos, yo soy de Nicaragua y estoy aprendiendo como funciona todo", dijo Camila.

"No fue nada. No te preocupes, siempre hay una primera vez para todo, y estoy encantada de ayudarte en lo que necesites", dijo Diana, segura de sí misma.

Un mes después de haber llegado a los Estados Unidos, Camila se empezó a sentir más cómoda. Batallaba un poco con el inglés, pero ella se quedó algunas veces después de la escuela con la señora Clay para que revisara su gramática. Para Camila, la señora Clay era como un ángel que había caído del cielo. Se preocupaba por ella. Regularmente le preguntaba si necesitaba algo, y la res-puesta de Camila siempre era la misma—ella necesitaba a su familia. Camila también practicaba el inglés con Diana, quien le caía bien a Camila. En Nicaragua, las cosas iban bien. Camila se aseguró de enviarle a su tía dinero para que siguiera cuidando de su familia. Charly extrañaba a Camila tanto como ella lo extrañaba a él, pero ahora tenía ropa nueva y siempre había comida en la mesa. Él sabía que su hermana trabajaba duro para enviar esos dólares, pero él quería estar con ella. Al igual que Camila, quería ir a los Estados Unidos, donde estaba su hermana mayor, la valiente. Un sábado por la noche, después de que Camila volviera del trabajo, Charly la llamó y le contó sobre sus planes.

"¡No, Charly!": Camila le gritó.

"¿Hasta que olvides de mí?!" Se hizo un silencio. La ira de Camila se volvieron lágrimas, "No digas eso. Yo nunca me olvidaría de ti Charly".

"Eso es lo que dices ahora", gritó.

"Escúchame, trataré de averiguar cómo podemos estar juntos en este lado. ¿De acuerdo?", ella dijo, tratando de pensar positivamente. "Pero, por favor, no me mientas y no hagas cosas sin yo saberlo primero. Charly, yo tuve mucha suerte. Si no hubiera sido por Melissa y Marco, yo no estaría aquí. Nadie hace lo que ellos hicieron por mí. Charly, a mí no me violaron, ni me golpearon. No quiero que te suceda nada malo, porque créeme, pueden suceder y suceden. Por favor, prométeme que no intentarás nada sin mi consentimiento" Camila le suplicó.

"Sólo si prometes que trataras de encontrar una manera de que todos podamos estar juntos" respondió Charly.

Al día siguiente, Camila se sentó en la clase pensando que ella no podía permitir que Charly viniera a los Estados Unidos solo. Al final de aquel día escolar, Camila habló con la señora Clay y ella le prometió que le iba a ayudar. Conocía a un buen abogado de inmigración, Mario, y fueron a hablar con él. Camila se sentía insegura y asustada.

Mario les propuso varias opciones. La abuela and Charly podrían solicitar una visa para obtener ayuda humanitaria, pero esto podría tomarse meses o años. Otra opción sería que ellos vinieran a los Estados Unidos ilegalmente y solicitaran ayuda una vez que estuvieran en el país. Todas las opciones sonaban arriesgadas—las solicitudes eran denegadas frecuentemente y los tribunales iban atrasados y se podía vivir años en el limbo. La última opción, la que más le gustaba a Camila era que ambos solicitaran una visa de turista. Cuando la visa de turista se venciera, podrían vivir como muchos otros en EE. UU. con un visado vencido—el abogado no habló de esa parte, pero Camila sabía.

Camila contactó a su tía y le informó sobre estas opciones. Estaba muy orgullosa de Camila por haber tomado ese papel tan grande y por ser valiente. Solicitaron la visa de turista y esperaron el día de las entrevistas.

La familia de Camila obtuvo la visa de turista en un plazo de tres meses. Habían pasado casi seis meses desde que Camila vio a su familia por última vez. Ella esperó en el áerea de llegadas del aeropuerto, y temblaba de emoción. Ella no podía creer como había cambiado su vida, era un cambio drástico, igualmente, la vida de su familia iba a cambiar drásticamente. Camila estaba cada vez más impaciente. De repente vio a un chico que llevaba una mochila y a dos mujeres que reconoció en seguida. "Mi familia", pensó. "Nunca más nos volveremos a separar", ella se dijo a sí misma mientras sus ojos encontraron los de las dos mujeres y las lágrimas recorrieron sus mejillas.

· 6 ·

ANA MARIA FORES TAMAYO

In her voluntary work with asylum seekers in Texas, writing the stories of cruelty she listens to in her work is a catharsis for Ana Maria Fores Tamayo. In this poem about a 7-year-old child, crimson colors reveal a haunting memory of rape and murder. The author, who was herself a child refugee, has heard similar stories of violence and displacement as the one told in this poem.

Elegy to a Refugee Girl

The teacher collected the young child's drawing.
Looking it over, she stared intently
at the little girl's work:
she saw
a young child, separated by bars.
a large splash of crimson covering the trees she had drawn.
A larger lady in the background faraway,
brown on brown her hair falling wildly
on the page,
so that all she could see
were splashes of sepia with a little green
but much more blood red.

the wild woman seen in the image
had something shackling her ankle,
her face blotched with droplets upon her cheeks.
What did you paint, sweetheart?
the teacher slowly questioned
the young child with the immense, sorrowful eyes.
And the girl looked up, giant eyes tearing,
voice quivering,
repeating softly--
my *mami*, she whispered.
my *mami* was taken away.
She flew to the trees there, to the blue in the sky.
She was put in that *cárcel*, you see?
but her spirit flew
like the birds when they soar through the sky, stormy yet safe.

And the teacher stared at the sanguine red, what seemed
to be the color of gore,
and again she gazed inquisitively at the child . . .

My *mami* is a rose,
and the wilderness in her spirit breaks free
as she wails for my *papi*, red blood screaming pain.

Me escondí, a stifled sigh to the teacher.
Tenía miedo . . .
I hid myself under the *cama*, the bed skirt muting
my silent shrieks
as I saw my *papi's* red *sangre* spilling from him.
I stayed still and quiet under that bed
afraid they would see me,
those ugly green suits
taking my *papi* and hitting him, again and again,
so that he
became a scarlet jumble of pain.

my *mami* had no time to react as those ugly men
took her and threw her on top of me . . .
they did not know I was hiding under the bed.
But my *mami* knew, and she tried to be still
as the beasts tore into her, they ripped off her clothes, I think,
they strangled her cries, they heaved themselves
on top of her.
First one, then the other. Then a third.

My *mami* did not move.
I sang blue songs in my head and listened to the fairy birds
ringing out their tune of love, of my *mami* and *papi*
and their love for me ...
It was a long time the men were there and my *mami* not moving.
But finally what seemed to hump and hump and hump again
stopped moving,
and the bad ugly men in their green army suits all splattered with red were gone.

I stayed under the *cama*, afraid to come out
afraid to have the red stain my hands, sink through my fingers.
so I crawled into myself, staying below.

But finally I felt some movement.
My *mami* came back from the skies
from the blue heavens with the *loros* singing ...
she did not leave me, she stayed that *rosa* in the ground
for her baby girl.
my *mami* stumbled almost falling.
She lowered her body
crawling beneath that *cama*,
holding me, closely, loving me, touching me to make sure I was real
flesh and bone and not the red of my father,
the body limp without movement.
His eyes -- I finally saw -- were open wide staring blankly
at nothing. No heaven was open to his
rust stained drip
spilling all over the floor.

I knew my *mami* was hurt.
I knew it was hard to walk
but we took off, my *mami* and me,
and we traveled the death roads for heaven
thinking if we made it to *el norte*, good people would see us and
gather us into their embrace.

How strange it is that I am here in a school while my *mami*
is jailed for a crime she never committed?
For being forced by some bad bad men and she only trying to save me?
Why is it that others do not see *mi dolor*, my *mami's* ache,
because I weep inside
like a salamander devastated by poison?

The teacher looked at my drawing again, then she looked at me.
I saw her face, too, blotched with droplets upon her cheeks ...

Why does she cry like my *mami*? And will I see my *mami* again?
Why do these ugly men -- now wearing blue suits instead of the green I despise --
take my *mami* away?
Why have they placed me in this *escuela*,
in this place with other sad children who
say nothing look at nothing feel nothing
because *ellos también tienen miedo*?

Please teacher, *maestra*, take me to my *mami*.
Don't let her cry alone, *por favor* . . .
Don't let her fly in that cell room forsaken,
let me be with my *mami*, please.
I don't want to learn English,
I don't want fine things *if* my *mami* is destroyed in your cell.
the young girl with the immense, sorrowful eyes
voiced long silent stabbings with her muted gaze.

You are killing me, *not* softly, *not* kindly, she uttered.

killing

      killing

            killing

                  killing

                        killing

Oda a una niña refugiada

La maestra recogía lo que había dibujado la niñita.
Al verlo, miró fijamente
el trabajo de su pupila:
observó en la página
una pequeña mocosa, separada del mundo por barras.
Una gran capa de carmesí cubriendo los árboles.
Una señora en el fondo lejano,
marrón contra marrón, su cabello salvajemente golpeando
la página.
Solo percibía
retazos de sepia con un poco de verde
y mucho más rojo de sangre.

La indómita mujer que contemplaba en la imagen
tenía un grillete encadenando su tobillo,
la cara manchada de lágrimas.

¿Qué pintaste, corazón?
La maestra preguntaba lentamente
a la pequeña pupila con unos ojos inmensos, tristes.
Y la chiquita levantaba su vista, ojos gigantes, sollozando,
su voz temblorosa
repitiendo suavemente--
mi mami . . . susurró.
Mi mami fue secuestrada.
Ella voló hacia los árboles allá, hacia el azul celeste del cielo.
A ella la metieron en esa *cárcel*, ¿entiende?
Pero su espíritu se escapó
como los pájaros cuando se elevan hacia el cielo, tempestuosos pero seguros.

Y la maestra contemplaba el rojo sangre, lo que parecía
ser un monstruoso derrame,
y una vez más miraba a la niña curiosamente . . .

Mi mami es una rosa, decía,
y el desierto en su espíritu se libera
mientras ella llora por mi papi, dolor de sangre y llantos.

Me escondí . . . susurró un sofocado suspiro a la maestra.
Tenía miedo . . .

Me escondí bajo la cama, las sábanas cubriendo
mis silenciosos gritos
al ver la sangre escarlata de mi papi.
Me quedé quieta quieta bajo esa cama enorme,
con miedo que me sospecharan,
esos feos trajes verdes
atrapando a mi papi y golpeándolo, una y otra vez,
mientras él
se convertía en un caos de sangre y pena.

Mi mami no tuvo tiempo de reaccionar cuando esos feos hombres
la tiraron encima de mí, la raptaron . . .
no sabían que yo estaba escondida bajo la cama.
Pero mi mami sí lo sabía, y ella se quedaba quieta quieta
cuando esas bestias le arrancaban la ropa, cuando se la clavaban,
le estrangulaban sus gritos, se lanzaban
encima de ella
Primero uno, luego el otro. Después, un tercero otra vez más.

Y mi mami no se movía.
En silencio, yo cantaba canciones azules y escuchaba a los pájaros,
entonando su melodía de amor, de mi mami y mi papi
y su amor por mí . . .

Pasó mucho tiempo con esos hombres allí mientras mi mami no se movía.
Finalmente, lo que parecía cascar y cascar y cascar otra vez
dejó de moverse,
y esos grotescos, sus trajes de ejército salpicados de rojo, desaparecieron.

Me quedé bajo la cama, con terror de salir,
con terror de mancharme las manos de sangre, ese rojizo de muerte hundiéndose
    entre mis dedos.
Hui dentro de mí, enterrándome en las tinieblas de la noche.

Pero finalmente sentí algo de movimiento.
Mi mami regresaba de los cielos,
desde ese horizonte azul con los loros cantando . . .
ella no me dejó, mi mami; se quedó como esa rosa en la tierra
con su hija adorada.
Sin embargo, se tropezaba, casi caía.
Agachaba su cuerpo,
arrastrándose debajo la cama,
y me sostenía cerquita, amándome, acariciándome, asegurándose que era real,
carne y hueso y no el rojo de mi papi,
su cuerpo sin movimiento.
Sus ojos - finalmente los vi - estaban abiertos, mirando fijamente
a la nada. Ningún cielo quedaba abierto a su
goteo infinito, manchado de óxido,
derramándose por el suelo de piedra.

Sabía que mi mami estaba herida.
Sabía que era difícil caminar
pero igual nos escapamos, mi mami y yo,
y viajamos por los caminos de la muerte hacia el cielo,
pensando que, si lográbamos llegar al norte, gente buena
siempre nos acogiera en su abrazo.

¡Qué extraño estando aquí en una escuela mientras mi mami
se encuentra en la cárcel por un crimen que no cometió!
Por haber sido violada y ella ¿solo tratando de salvarme?
¿Por qué es que los demás no ven mi dolor, el dolor de mi madre?
¿Por qué lloro dentro
como una salamandra herida por un veneno siniestro?

La maestra contemplaba mi dibujo, y luego me miraba.
   Yo notaba su cara también, sus mejillas manchadas de lágrimas ...

¿Por qué llora la maestra igual que mi mami? ¿Y volveré a ver a mi mami?
¿Por qué esos feos -- ahora de azul en lugar del verde que odio --
atrapan a mi mami y se la llevan lejos de mi?
¿Por qué me han puesto en este frío colegio,
en este lugar con otros tristes niños que
no dicen nada, no miran nada, no sienten nada
porque ellos también tienen miedo?
Por favor maestra, *teacher*, lléveme a mi mami.
No la deje llorar sola, *oh please* ...
No la deje volar abandonada en la celda,
déjeme estar con mi mami, le ruego.
No quiero aprender inglés,
No quiero cosas buenas si mi mami cae destruida en su celda.

la niña con los ojos tristes e inmensos
anunciaba agotados silencios
apuñalando esa mirada apagada.

Me están matando, decía. No suavemente, no cariñosamente.
Me están ...

asesinando

                    asesinando

                              asesinando

                                        asesinando

                                                  asesinando

Part III
SILENCING

7

MARIA BAÑOS JORDAN

For Baños Jordan, linguistic and cultural barriers impact girls' willingness to speak up and the ability to develop connections. Schools are ill-prepared to work with transitional communities, often with staff who is not diverse or not trained in diversity. For instance, they might not know how to work with different gender expectations in Latin America. Most young women have been taught not to be opinionated. In the workshops where she participated with Latina professionals, middle-school newcomers expressed the sense of exclusion from the school culture, the teasing from non-Latino classmates, the lack of compassion from some adults, and their anxieties about their parents' struggle with poverty and legal status.

Spanish Silencio

You call me shy, but it's not me.
I am the dancer, the singer, the storyteller.
I am the dreamer soaring high above tall pines.
My lips tightened long ago, when I chose to speak mostly through my big brown eyes.
When my first words began to flow too freely, too loudly,
The elders captured them, and stitched them with string

To the hem of my dress where they dangled like lace.
My thoughts are much older now in this other land,
But my tongue fails me with the words I don't know, that I don't feel,
So I keep it short, sweet, and smile a lot.
You tilt your head waiting for my stories,
But they won't dare leave the Spanish warmth of my mind.
Words fail me, and then I will fail you,
So I keep my *silencio* knowing you can't judge what you can't hear.
We both know it's there- the veil between two worlds,
But maybe you'll still accept me,
Maybe you'll meet me within the space beyond the veil . . .
Where you'll find my true spirit,
Longing to fly without strings,
Longing to be known.

Silencio
Wendy Herrera (Translator)

Me llamas tímida, pero no lo soy yo.
Soy bailarina, cantante, narradora.
Soy la soñadora que se eleva por encima de los pinos altos.
Mis labios se sellaron hace mucho tiempo, cuando decidí expresarme por medio de mis
    grandes ojos marrones.
Cuando mis primeras palabras empezaron a fluir libre y fuertemente,
los ancianos las capturaron, y las cosieron con hilo
al dobladillo de mi vestido, donde colgaron como encaje.
Ahora en esta tierra, mis pensamientos ya son mucho más viejos,
pero mi lengua me falla con las palabras que no sé, que no siento,
por eso, hablo poco, breve, y sonrío mucho.
Inclinas la cabeza esperando que te cuente,
pero no se atreverán a dejar salir el calor español de mi mente.
Las palabras me fallan, y por eso te fallaré,
así las aguardo en mi silencio, sabiendo que no las puedes juzgar porque no las oyes.
Ambos sabemos que están allí, en el velo entre dos mundos,
pero tal vez todavía me aceptes,
tal vez me encontrarás en el espacio más allá del velo . . .
Donde encontrarás mi verdadero espíritu,
anhelando volar sin cuerdas,
anhelando ser conocida.

8

FRANCISCO VILLEGAS
AND PALOMA VILLEGAS

F. Villegas and P. Villegas describe their own schooling experience in the 1990s. As undocumented children, school felt like a psychological border built on the stressors emanating from the fears about deportation, proper access to resources, and bullying.

Reflection on Schooling Experiences as Undocumented Migrants in the U.S.

The poem and image by Paloma Villegas published in this anthology illustrate the crossing of borders without state required documents. This narrative focuses on the last two stanzas of the poem that detail the processes through which borders encrust themselves onto our bodies. One way to think through that process is through the concept of internal borders: borders that extend beyond the geographic delineation of nation-states and impact migrants as they go through their day-to-day lives.[1] More specifically, we focus on one internal border: schooling. Schooling is often considered the great equalizer, the "meritocratic" structure that will facilitate social mobility and financial stability. However, the intersections of race, gender, class, and immigration status serve as significant barriers to realizing this dream.

We were born in Mexico and arrived in the U.S. at the ages of 11 and 8. This was the early 1990s California, when anti-immigrant rhetoric manifested itself openly with policies such as Proposition 187. Upon our arrival, Francisco enrolled in the 7th grade and Paloma in the 4th grade. We always knew we were undocumented, however, understanding the consequences of this classification came in stages, acquired piece-meal, as "nuggets" of information every time we were ineligible to do something considered age-appropriate.

From an early age, we learned to fear the request for documents, including a social security number. It meant rejection and danger. While the Supreme Court decision Plyler v. Doe guarantees access to K-12 schooling for undocumented children, undocumented migrants know there is a difference between policy and practice. This is where a nuanced meaning for access is required. Access is not only getting through a door; it is feeling welcomed and having the opportunity to participate in a community. This sense of belonging was affected by our recognition of deportability and the fear it produced.[2] Fear was not only constrained to our subjective understanding of safety, but it was also enhanced by input from family members, stories heard in the news, and lack of knowledge about the legal and social entitlements to which undocumented migrants had access. This is not to imply that our fear was unfounded, rather, the context of precarity facilitated the circulation of multiple fears that could not be dispelled. In terms of our schooling, the exclusions we faced meant an inability to receive free lunch, attend a school trip, or engage in school activities.

Those consequences were also applied differently between us. For example, Francisco was often left behind during school trip days. Our mother chose this option given the family's lack of funds and stories about kids getting hurt and needing to go to the doctor where they would be asked for insurance or about kids traveling across international boundaries and not allowed to return. When people asked him questions about not attending a free trip, he answered that his mother was mad at him, or that she did not trust a particular teacher. As a result, he had to sit in the main office with nothing to do because no other adult was available to supervise him. While these days were filled with boredom and longing, what he remembers most is the anxiety. An overwhelming concern that his status would be readily apparent to people around and that his family would be deported. Paloma did not have those experiences. She encountered generous teachers who paid for her school trips, even taking her camping, never once having to provide a social security number.

While immigration status was a salient facet of our schooling trajectory, it is impossible to disentangle it from race and class. Both factors led Francisco to hate lunch time. Given our social status, as well as our cultural capital, our mother made us lunches as best she could. Usually, this meant refried bean sandwiches with a little mayonnaise or mustard, so they would not be too dry. These were the epitome of poverty and racialization in Francisco's school and in addition to his awkwardness, resulted in being increasingly ostracized. When his peers asked why he did not buy lunch from the cafeteria he learned to respond that he did not want nasty food, while salivating at their meals. Our mother, not understanding the effects of race in schooling in the U.S. and rightfully proud of being able to feed her children, did not understand when Francisco returned home with uneaten sandwiches. Obviously, this experience is not only caused by immigration status. Many children of immigrants and working-class students face social stigma for not assimilating to the normative U.S. lunch: ham or peanut butter and jelly sandwiches. However, immigration status framed Francisco's understanding of the situation.

Food was also important for Paloma. In elementary school, she was selected to deliver hot lunches to other classrooms. While this was a process of exploiting children's labor, Paloma felt proud, for her payment was that she could also partake of a hot school lunch, for free. The message was once again one of assimilation and a rejection of bean sandwiches. And yet, those bean and mustard sandwiches are what she longingly thinks about when she thinks about food from that time.

When she first arrived in the fourth grade, there was a white female student who bullied Paloma during recess and stepped on her feet. This was not a quick tap, but a hard, repeated, thump, every day for months. Paloma had a difficult time responding to the aggression. She did not yet know English, and she froze whenever the young girl approached. When she finally told her mother and aunt, the latter told her to say, "Stop it!" However, the response did not garner the hope for change. And, while her mother was concerned, she felt helpless, unable to go to the school and report the child because of her lack of English proficiency and her immigration status.

Trouble with language was a constant and included being excluded from the learning environment, having to learn to act as interpreters, and others reading our accent as a deficiency. Upon arrival, Francisco's school did not have an ESL program or bilingual instructors, aside from Spanish teachers. Francisco quickly learned that classroom expectations were to remain silent and invisible. There has been a large amount of literature detailing the immigrant paradox in schooling, specifically that migrant students often outperform their locally born peers initially and gradually see their grades drop.[3] Although in Mexico he had excelled academically, Francisco struggled in school. As an English learner, English class was a mystery to him, he could not read the literature assigned or partake in conversations about the stories, and he was excluded from group work. In History class, it took over a month to receive a textbook and he relied on pictures to develop a reading of the material. Finally, Math and Science, once his strong suit did not provide an entry point to engage. Altogether this led to barely passing that year. A mentor could have ameliorated some of these effects, but no one would be found that year, though they were available in the eighth grade. Instead, school felt like a foreign place, one where Francisco embodied the visitor, one to be tolerated but summarily dismissed with nothing to offer and little being offered. Paloma had a similar experience. She had an ESL tutor who came in once a week and taught her how to say words like "airplane" using picture cards. Although useful, this information did not help her understand her course work. Nonetheless, her experience was tempered by her younger age, and the fact that grades did not matter as much in elementary school.

Another experience relating to language involved the reading of our accent as a deficiency, which numerous people recommended us to "overcome." Teachers saw our accent as a challenge, something to remove before it was too late, lest it remain for a lifetime. As a result, we both remember being praised at signs of its loss. While we were proud to have learned English quickly, it was not until later that we understood the violence enacted in such comments, both externally by educators as well as internally by feeling proud of the increased distance from this signifier of "deficiency." Paloma also received recommendations from white immigrants who had lost their accents to keep ours. They did not understand the hierarchy of privilege that derives from having or not having a Latinx accent.

Finally, like many children of immigrants, we were often tasked with interpreting for our mother. Because of her precarious employment as a housecleaner and her limited English, she was only able to attend one student-teacher conference for Paloma, during the sixth grade. Even though she was a good student, it was an uncomfortable experience explaining her accomplishments and shortcomings. The teacher at one point noted a grade of Satisfactory, as opposed to Excellent, for a particular component of her evaluation, which made Paloma feel bad and tear up. Her mother, not understanding what was going on, also teared up. Discussions of immigrant parents not caring about their children's schooling circulate in academic scholarship and public discourse, but negative representations reproduce deficiency theories that are both false and violent.[4] As Paloma's experience demonstrates, despite her language limitations, the mother found the child's schooling experience important for the mother, she was affectively and physically invested in it.

The undocumented experience for us was filled with social isolation, particularly when we knew that any person could act like an immigration agent and that there is a multiplicative effect linked to the danger of immigration enforcement. Hence, safety meant being quiet. Safety meant the ability to think quickly and find a reason as to why we could not engage in school activities, whether by peers or educators. Being quiet produced a degree of seclusion. Thus, our undocumented experience was filled with fear and anxiety. It meant the need to describe our subjectivity in ways that would remove suspicions about our status and avoid "uncomfortable questions." From an early age, we made a family pact to not disclose our status. Gloria Anzaldúa described the borderlands as a subjectivity that simultaneously merges and divides, a space of continuous tension.[5] Our childhood in the borderlands was one of multiple exclusions and possible expulsion. The struggle of hoping to achieve the "American dream" occurred knowing that our very presence was precarious and through it all, struggling with the seduction of assimilation. Mainly, unable to speak about our undocumented experience with any peers was isolating. And this feeling, like the poem describes, persists well into adulthood. Finally, the *florero* is an important metaphor. As displaced individuals suffering constant precarity, our roots remained firm and well built in us, while they were also quite fluid. Home expanded beyond a geographic space, and we carried it within us.

Una reflexión sobre nuestra propia escolarización como migrantes indocumentados en los EE. UU.
Montse Feu (Translator)

El poema y la ilustración que Paloma Villegas publica en esta colección ejemplariza el cruzar de fronteras sin los documentos estatales requeridos. Este ensayo se centra en las dos últimas estrofas del poema que detallan los procesos por lo cuales las fronteras se incrustan en nuestros cuerpos. Un modo de pensar tales procesos es mediante el concepto de la frontera interna. Aquellas que se extienden más allá de la delineación geográfica de las naciones-estado e impactan migrantes mientras llevan a cabo el día a día. En concreto, nos enfocamos en una frontera interna específica: la escolarización. La escolarización se considera a menudo la gran manera de igualar en una estructura de meritocracia que facilitará el ascenso social y la estabilidad financiera. Sin embargo, la intersección de la racialización, el género, la clase social y el estatus migratorio son barreras significativas para que se haga realidad el sueño americano.

Nacimos en México y llegamos a los Estados Unidos cuando teníamos once y ocho años. Estábamos en California, al principio de los 1990s, cuando la retórica antiinmigrante se manifestaba abiertamente con políticas tales como la Proposition 187. En cuanto llegamos, Francisco se registró en el séptimo grado y Paloma en el cuarto. Siempre supimos que éramos indocumentados, sin embargo, el entendimiento de las consecuencias de tal clasificación vino poco a poco, a pedazos, como si trocitos de información cada vez que no teníamos derecho a participar en actividades de nuestra edad.

Desde pequeños aprendimos a temer posibles peticiones de documentación, incluyendo el número de la seguridad social. Significaba rechazo y peligro. Mientras que la decisión de la Corte Suprema Plyler v. Doe garantiza acceso a K-12 para los niños indocumentados, los inmigrados saben que existe una diferencia entre política y práctica. Ahí radical el significado sutil del acceso real, que no significa entrar por una puerta, sino sentirse bienvenido y tener las mismas oportunidades de participar en la comunidad. Nuestro conocimiento de poder ser deportados afectó negativamente este sentido de pertenencia y produjo miedo. El miedo no estaba restringido a nuestro entendimiento de seguridad, sino que se reforzaba con las aportaciones de nuestros familiares, las historias que escuchábamos en las noticias y la falta de conocimiento de los derechos legales y sociales a que los inmigrados indocumentados pueden acceder. Esto no implica que nuestro miedo no estuviera fundamentado, sino que el contexto precario facilitaba que la multiplicación de miedos no se dispersara. En cuanto a nuestra escolarización, la exclusión que sufrimos fue que no recibimos almuerzo gratuito, no asistimos a las excursiones escolares, ni participamos de ciertas actividades escolares.

Estas consecuencias también se aplicaron de modo distinto entre nosotros. Por ejemplo, Francisco no iba a las excursiones escolares. Nuestra madre así lo decidió a causa de la falta de recursos y por lo que había escuchado sobre los niños podían hacerse daño y ser llevados al médico donde se le pediría por el seguro médico o sobre los niños cruzando fronteras que luego les impedirían volver. Cuando la gente le preguntaba sobre su asistencia a una excursión gratuita, contestaba que su madre no dejaba porque se había portado mal o que no confiaba con un maestro en particular. En consecuencia, tenía que pasarse el tiempo sentado en la oficina principal sin nada que hacer porque no había adultos que lo pudieran supervisar. Aunque estos días eran aburridos y largos, lo que más recuerda es la ansiedad. Una preocupación abrumadora de que su estatus migratorio sería fácilmente aparente y que su familia sería deportada. Paloma no sufrió estas experiencias. Tuvo maestros generosos que pagaron sus excursiones, incluso se la llevaron de acampada, y nunca tuvo que dar un número de la seguridad social.

Mientras que el estado migratorio fue una faceta destacada de nuestra escolarización, es imposible separarlo de nuestra racialización y clase social. Ambos factores hicieron que Francisco odiase la hora del almuerzo. Por nuestro estatus social y capital cultural, nuestra madre nos hacía los mejores almuerzos que podía. Normalmente, esto significaba emparedados de frijoles refritos con mayonesa o mostaza para que no estuvieran muy secos. Eran el paradigma de pobreza y racialización en la escuela de Francisco. Además, por la vergüenza que pasaba, aun lo excluían más. Cuando sus compañeros le preguntaban por qué no compraba almuerzo en la cafetería, aprendió a contestar que no quería comida basura, pero salivaba por sus comidas. Nuestra madre, quien no entendía los efectos de la racialización en la escuela norteamericana y estaba legítimamente orgullosa de poder alimentar a sus hijos, no entendía cuando Francisco volvía a casa sin haber comido sus emparedados. Obviamente, esta experiencia no es causa exclusivamente del estatus migratorio. Muchos hijos de inmigrantes y de trabajadores sufren el estigma social por no asimilarse a las expectativas de un almuerzo norteamericano: emparedados de jamón o de manteca d cacauetes y mermelada. Aún así, el estatus migratorio de Francisco enmarcaba su entendimiento de la situación.

La comida también fue importante para Paloma. En la escuela primaria, fue seleccionada para distribuir los almuerzos calientes en otras clases. Aunque se trataba de cierta explotación infantil, Paloma se sentía orgullosa de hacerlo y además como pago podía comer una comida caliente. Así, otra vez se repetía el mensaje de que la asimilación llevaba consigo el rechazo de los emparedados de frijoles. Sin embargo, son esos emparedados de frijoles lo que recuerda con anhelo cuando piensa en la comida de ese tiempo. Cuando estaba en cuarto grado, una estudiante blanca la seguía en recreo y le pisaba los pies. No se trataba de un golpecito sino de golpes repetidos cada día durante meses. Paloma no sabía como responder a tal agresión. No sabía inglés, y se paralizaba cada vez que la niña se le acercaba. Cuando por fin se lo dijo a su madre y a su

tía, ésta le recomendó que le dijera, "¡Basta!" Esa respuesta no le dio le esperanza de cambiar. Aunque su madre estaba preocupada, se sentía indefensa, sin
poder ir a la escuela y informar sobre lo sucedido por su falta de dominio del
inglés y su estatus migratorio.

Los problemas con el idioma fueron constantes e incluyeron la exclusión
del entorno de aprendizaje, el aprender a actuar como interpretes, y la lectura
de otros de nuestro acento como deficiencia. Cuando Francisco llegó a los
Estados Unidos, su escuela no tenía un programa ESL ni instructores bilingües
que no fueran maestros de español. Francisco pronto aprendió que lo que se
esperaba de él era que estuviera callado e invisible en clase. Se ha publicado
mucho sobre la paradoja del inmigrante en la educación, en particular como
algunos estudiantes migrantes con frecuencia consiguen mejores resultados
que sus compañeros de escuela nacidos en Estados Unidos pero sus calificaciones empeorar paulatinamente. Aunque en México, se había distinguido
académicamente, a Francisco le costó en Estados Unidos. Como aprendiz de
inglés, le resultaba un misterio el idioma, no podía leer las lecturas asignadas
en clase o conversar sobre ellas en clase y se le excluía del trabajo en grupo.
En la clase de historia, pasó más de un mes hasta que recibió el libro de texto
e incluso entonces tuvo que confiar en las fotos para interpretar el material.
Por último, las matemáticas y la ciencia, que habían sido sus materias fuertes,
no le sirvieron para involucrarse. Con todo esto, apenas aprobó ese año. Un
mentor hubiera podido mejorar estos efectos, no se pudo encontrar ninguno
eso año, a pesar de haberlos en el grado octavo. Por ello la escuela era como un
lugar extranjero, en el cual Francisco personificaba el visitante, a aquel que se
toleraba, pero que sumariamente se le despachaba con poco o nada que ofre-
cerle. Paloma tuvo una experiencia similar. Tuvo un tutor de ESL una vez por
semana que le enseñó a decir palabras como "airplane" con tarjetas ilustradas.
Si bien fue útil, esta información no le ayudó a entender las materias. De todos
modos, su experiencia estuvo mitigada por su temprana edad y por el hecho
que las calificaciones no eran tan importantes en la escuela primaria.

Otra experiencia relacionada con el idioma fue el entendimiento de otros
de nuestro acento como una deficiencia, que mucha gente nos recomendó
que superásemos. Los maestros percibían nuestro acento como un reto, algo
que había que eliminar antes de que fuera demasiado tarde, por temor de que
permaneciera una vida entera. Como resultado, recordamos ser elogiados en
cuanto mostrábamos señales de su pérdida. Mientras que estábamos orgullosos
de haber aprendido inglés rápidamente, no fue hasta más tarde que enten-
dimos la violencia ejercida en tales comentarios, tanto por aquellos de los

educadores como aquellos que internamente nos decíamos orgullosos de la creciente distancia a un significante de "deficiencia." Paloma a su vez recibió recomendaciones de inmigrantes blancos que habían perdido sus acentos de que nosotros no perdiéramos el nuestro. Esas personas no entendían la jerarquía de privilegio que se deriva de tener o no tener acento.

Finalmente, como muchos hijos de inmigrantes, frecuentemente se nos pedía que interpretáramos para nuestra madre. A causa de su empleo precario como personal de limpieza y su inglés limitado, solo pudo atender una reunión con la profesora de Paloma, en el sexto grado. Aunque era una buena estudiante, le fue incómodo explicar sus logros y posibilidades de mejora. En un momento dado, la profesora mencionó que su calificación sería Satisfactoria y no Excelente, a causa de un componente específico de la evaluación. Ello causó que Paloma se sintiera mal y se le llenasen los ojos de lágrimas. Su madre, que no entendía que estaba pasando, también se puso a llorar. Debates sobre la preocupación de los padres inmigrantes por la escolarización de sus hijos circulan en la investigación académica, pero representaciones negativas reproducen teorías de deficiencia que son falsas y violentas. Como la experiencia de Paloma demuestra, a pesar de sus limitaciones en el idioma, su madre consideraba importante la experiencia de su hija y física y mentalmente se involucraba en ella.

Nuestra experiencia indocumentada estuvo llena de aislamiento social, especialmente cuando sabíamos que cualquier persona podía actuar como un agente de inmigración y por tanto había un efecto multiplicador del peligro del cuerpo de inmigración. De ahí que, la seguridad radicaba en permanecer callado. La seguridad significaba la capacidad de pensar rápido, y decir una razón por la que no podíamos participar en actividades escolares, ya fueran de compañeros o de educadores. El estar callado produjo un nivel de reclusión. Así, nuestra experiencia indocumentada estaba llena de ansiedad. Significaba describir nuestra subjetividad en modos que eliminaran cualquier sospecha sobre nuestro estado migratorio y evitara preguntas incómodas. Desde muy jóvenes, hicimos un pacto de no revelar nuestro estado migratorio. Gloria Anzaldúa describió la frontera como una subjetividad que a la vez une y divide, un espacio de tensión continuada. Nuestra niñez en la frontera fue una de muchas exclusiones y de posible expulsión. La lucha de desear conseguir el sueño americano ocurrió mientras sabíamos que nuestra presencia era precaria y que, todo el tiempo, luchábamos con la seducción de la asimilación. Principalmente, el no poder hablar sobre nuestra condición de indocumentados con los compañeros nos apartó. Este sentimiento, como el poema describe, persiste aún en nuestra edad adulta. Finalmente, el florero es una metáfora importante. Como individuos desarraigados que han sufrido constante precariedad, nuestras raíces se mantienen firmes y bien encastradas en nosotros, aunque seamos bien fluidos. Nuestro hogar se extendió más allá del espacio geográfico y lo transportamos con nosotros.

Notes

1. Mutsaers, Paul. "An Ethnographic Study of the Policing of Internal Borders of the Netherlands," *British Journal of Criminology* 54, no. 5 (2014): 831–48.
2. De Genova, Nicholas P. "Migrant 'Illegality' and Deportability in Everyday Life," *Annual Review of Anthropology* 31 (2002): 419–47.
3. Suárez-Orozco, Carola, Jean Rhodes, and Michael Milburn. "Unraveling the Immigrant Paradox: Academic Engagement and Disengagement Among Recently Arrived Immigrant Youth," *Youth and Society* 41, no. 2 (2009): 151–85.
4. Villegas, Francisco. "Prescribe Lack: The Prevalence and Dangers of Deficiency Theories to Explain the Latina/o Schooling Experience in Toronto," *Latin American Encounters* 2 (2014): 40–50.
5. Anzaldúa, Gloria. *Borderlands/la frontera: The New Mestiza* (2nd ed.). San Francisco: Aunt Lute Books, 1999.

References

Anzaldúa, Gloria. *Borderlands/la frontera: The New Mestiza* (2nd ed.). San Francisco: Aunt Lute Books. 1999

Creswell, John W., and Cheryl N. Poth. *Qualitative Inquiry & Research Design: Choosing Among Five Approaches* (4th ed.). Thousand Oaks: Sage Publications, Inc., 2018.

De Genova, Nicholas P. "Migrant 'Illegality' and Deportability in Everyday Life," *Annual Review of Anthropology* 31 (2002): 419–47.

Mateo, José Manuel. *Migrant: The Journey of a Mexican Worker.* New York: Abrams Books, 2014.

Meretoja, Hanna. *The Ethics of Storytelling. Narrative Hermeneutics, History, and the Possible.* New York: Oxford University Press, 2018.

Mutsaers, Paul. "An Ethnographic Study of the Policing of Internal Borders of the Netherlands," *British Journal of Criminology* 54, no. 5 (2014): 831–48.

Villegas, Francisco. "Prescribe Lack: The Prevalence and Dangers of Deficiency Theories to Explain the Latina/o Schooling Experience in Toronto," *Latin American Encounters* 2 (2014): 40–50.

· 9 ·

ESTRELLA GODINEZ

Godinez conducted interviews with Central American newcomers and their caregivers in a school for immigrant youth in Texas from 2016 to 2018. A refugee advocate, Godinez has noticed how religion is a recurrent theme. Faith gives strength to Latinos. She tells the inspiring story of Danny Mateo, who she witnesses fighting for a better life.

A Yearning Desire

All day Danny Mateo sold individual pieces of candy in Temascalcingo, Mexico and at night he witnessed his mother become the victim of his father's alcoholism. He dreamt of a perfect family. One dreary night, his sister Rosario didn't come home, but sent Danny Mateo a note with her boyfriend, Tacho, saying "Danny by the time you read this I will be far gone. I don't know if I will make it across the border, but I am taking this risk for my baby. I will never tell him I was raped by my own father. But I will tell him that I wanted him to have a life free of violence. And I want the same for you. I left you some money with Tacho and he will give it to you when you are ready to leave Temascalcingo. I saved enough money for the two of us by working late nights. I hope to see you on the other side."

One night, Danny Mateo said to his mother, "Mother, I don't want to leave you alone. Rosario had her own reasons to leave but I could never abandon you." His mom said to him, "Mateo do not be afraid, I want the best for you. I want you to work and go to school, become a nurse, and help others with the caring heart that God has given you. I know you have a purpose in life, so go find it." He looked for his red cloth that had rubber bands wrapped around it. Once he found it, he opened it to count his change that he had saved while selling candy. He walked to his mother with a frown on his face. "*Mamá* look at this, this isn't enough." His mother reached into her blouse and took out a small handmade wooden cross. She blessed him and said, "Son, I've been saving this for you. Take it and hold it tight along the way. And remember that our heavenly father is always by your side."

Danny Mateo decided to leave Temascalcingo and go to America at age fifteen, carrying a small backpack on his shoulders. Tacho took him to an older man who was known for crossing people successfully from Mexico to the United States. Tacho handed the man a wad of money that Rosario had given him specifically for her brother. After a 13-hour ride, Danny Mateo arrived at the U.S. border, he knew that crossing would be dangerous, so he followed detailed instructions from the older man. He was told to get under an eighteen-wheeler truck and to fit his body into a small section. Danny Mateo hung on tightly as they crossed into the U.S.

A truck driver told Danny Mateo that he could only take him directly to Victoria if he paid him extra money. Impulsively, he emptied his bag with only the wooden cross his mother had given him, and about ten dollars. The truck driver dropped him off at the nearest town of Kingsville, apparently without a second thought. Danny Mateo looked around him, he noticed big colorful signs. He could read some signs like "1.88 per gallon" and "Burger." He paid close attention to a sign outside a red brick church, "Today May 5, 2004 Jesus loves you and tomorrow he will love you once more." Danny Mateo recognized the word "Jesus" and made his way towards the church. A young American couple approached him. As good Samaritans they offered him a place to stay for the night. Little did he know that the couple would have a big influence in his life.

Danny Mateo spoke to his mother and his sister the next day. He told his sister he would work, for the time being, in order to save up enough money to make it to Victoria. He soon found a job as a dish washer and started working every night. He later became a server. At the same time, he began attending high school for English language learners. During his Junior year of high school, Danny Mateo signed up for Cosmetology. Although he was the only boy in the course, he realized he had found something he really liked. The course allowed him to meet new people and to use his creativity to style hair. He was always very social and talkative, and this career felt like a good fit for him. Being around women was normal for him—having grown up with mostly his mother and sister—and he got along well with the rest of his peers in Cosmetology. He knew that once he graduated, he could start working at a hair salon right away. But things did not go as Danny Mateo planned. He failed his state board exam on his first attempt. Defeated by the language barrier and was disappointed in himself, he felt as if his dreams would never come true. Stella, a friend from the Cosmetology program, encouraged him to keep studying for his licensing examination. Danny Mateo retook the exam four times before he finally passed. When Stella heard the news, she offered him a job at a local salon. He started to build up a clientele and saved enough money for his first car. Maybe he would be able to move to Victoria and live with his sister.

Meanwhile, Stella helped him enroll in a community college and select nursing classes, as he and his mother had always wanted for him. His English was better, but he still struggled. He felt overwhelmed and avoided calling home; he had nothing good to say. He felt embarrassed of his failures.

A Christian group that Danny Mateo had met at college sought him out. During worship, Danny Mateo had a revelation through prayer where he felt the presence of the Holy Spirit. The revelation was so powerful that he started to cry uncontrollably. It was revealed to him that one day he would be helping others with his nursing career and that he was not facing these obstacles alone. It was clear to him now that God was always by his side. He had crossed the border and had a bed to sleep the night he arrived in a new country. He finally understood the signs that God was sending him to show His unconditional love. He was finally doing well as a nursing student and became the leader of a religious youth group. Although Danny Mateo had to live away from his sister and mother, he learned to value the opportunities he was offered in the United States.

Un deseo anhelante

Cada mañana Danny Mateo vendía dulces en Temascalcingo, México y por la noche era testigo de cómo su madre era víctima del alcoholismo de su padre. Soñaba con una familia perfecta. Una noche triste, su hermana Rosario no fue a casa, pero mandó una nota por medio de su novio, Tacho, que decía "Danny cuando leas esto estaré lejos. No sé si lograré cruzar la frontera, pero estoy tomando este riesgo por mi bebé. Sí, estoy embarazada y quiero darle a mi hijo una vida mejor de la que llevamos aquí. No le diré nunca que fui violada por mi propio padre. Pero le diré que sí quise que tuviera una vida libre de violencia. Y quiero lo mismo para ti. He dejado algo de dinero con Tacho y él te lo dará cuando estés listo para irte de Temascalcingo. Ahorré suficiente dinero para los dos trabajando por las noches. Espero que entiendas mi sacrificio. Espero verte en el otro lado".

Una noche, Danny Mateo le dijo a su madre: "Madre, no quiero dejarte sola. Rosario tuvo sus propias razones para irse, pero yo nunca podría abandonarte". Su mamá le dijo, "Mateo no tengas miedo, quiero lo mejor para ti. Quiero que trabajes y que vayas a la escuela, y seas un enfermero y ayudes a otros con ese corazón que Dios te ha dado. Sé que tienes un propósito en la vida, ve y encuéntralo". Danny Mateo buscó el paño rojo que tenía amarrado con ligas. Una vez que lo encontró, lo abrió para contar las monedas que había ahorrado mientras vendía dulces. Él caminó hacia su madre con una mirada triste, "Mira mamá, esto no es suficiente", su madre sacó del pecho una pequeña cruz de madera hecha a mano. Ella lo bendijo y le dijo: "hijo, yo he estado guardando esto para ti. Tómalo y sostenlo firmemente en el camino. Y recuerda que nuestro Padre celestial estará siempre a tu lado".

Danny Mateo decidió dejar Temascalcingo e irse a los Estados Unidos a los quince años, con tan solo una pequeña mochila en sus hombros. Tacho lo llevó con un hombre mayor que era conocido por cruzar personas de México a los Estados Unidos con éxito. Tacho le dio al hombre un buen fajo de dinero que Rosario le había dado específicamente para su hermano. Después de un viaje de trece horas, Danny Mateo llegó a la frontera, él sabía que cruzar era peligroso así que él siguió las instrucciones de aquel hombre. Le dijeron que se acomodara debajo de un camión de dieciocho ruedas y que metiera su cuerpo en una pequeña sección. Danny Mateo se agarró fuerte mientras cruzaban la frontera.

Un conductor del camión le dijo a Danny Mateo que podría llevarlo directamente a Victoria si le pagaba un dinero extra. Impulsivamente vació su bolsa, pero sólo tenía la cruz de madera y alrededor de diez dólares. El conductor del camión lo dejó en la ciudad más cercana a Kingsville sin ningún remordimiento. Danny Mateo miró a su alrededor, vio grandes anuncios de colores y pudo leer "1.88 per gallon" y "Burger". Le llamó la atención un letrero fuera de una iglesia de ladrillo rojo que decía, "Today May 5, 2004 Jesus loves you and tomorrow he will love you once more". Danny Mateo reconoció la palabra "Jesús" y fue hacia la iglesia. Una pareja joven americana se le acercó. Como buenos samaritanos le ofrecieron un lugar para quedarse esa noche.

Danny Mateo habló con su madre y su hermana al día siguiente. Le dijo a su hermana que trabajaría de momento para ahorrar dinero para poder llegar a Victoria. Pronto encontró trabajo de lavaplatos en un restaurante cercano y más tarde se convirtió en un mesero. Durante su tercer año de preparatoria, se inscribió en cosmetología. Aunque él era el único niño en el curso, se dio cuenta de que había encontrado algo que realmente le gustaba. El curso le permitió conocer a gente nueva y a utilizar su creatividad para peinar. Siempre fue muy sociable y hablador y esta carrera la sentía perfecta para él. Era normal para él estar rodeado de mujeres, puesto que había crecido con su mamá y su hermana y se llevaba muy bien con todas sus compañeras de cosmetología. Sabía que una vez obtuviera su grado, podría empezar a trabajar en una peluquería en seguida pero las cosas no sucedieron como las había planeado. Danny Mateo reprobó su examen de cosmetología del estado en su primer intento. Derrotado por la barrera idiomática y decepcionado de sí mismo, se sentía como si sus sueños nunca se harían realidad. Stella, una amiga del programa de cosmetología, lo animó a seguir estudiando para su licencia. Le tomó cuatro veces tomarlo hasta que al final aprobó. Cuando Stella oyó la noticia, ella le ofreció un trabajo en un salón local. Danny Mateo era siempre puntual y estaba agradecido por la oportunidad. Comenzó a tener su propia clientela. Quizás podría ahorrar para ir a Victoria con su hermana.

Stella le ayudó a inscribirse en un colegio comunitario y empezó enfermería. Era lo que su madre siempre había querido para él. Su inglés mejoraba, pero aún batallaba. Se sentía abrumado y evitaba llamar a casa; no tenía nada bueno que decir. Le daban vergüenza los errores que cometía. Un grupo cristiano que Danny Mateo había conocido en la universidad lo visitó. Durante la adoración, Danny Mateo tuvo una revelación a través de la oración donde sintió la presencia del Espíritu Santo. La revelación fue tan poderosa que comenzó a llorar incontrolablemente. Se le fue revelado que un día él ayudaría a los demás con su carrera de enfermería, pero lo más importante es que no iba a superar los obstáculos solo. Estaba claro ahora que Dios siempre estaría con él. Cruzó la frontera y tuvo una cama donde dormir la noche que llegó a un nuevo país. Finalmente entendió las señales que Dios le enviaba para mostrarle su amor incondicional. Empezó a irle bien como un estudiante de enfermería y se convirtió en líder de un grupo religioso para jóvenes. Aunque Danny Mateo tenía que vivir lejos de su hermana y de su madre, aprendió a valorar las oportunidades que Estados Unidos le ofrecía.

· 1 0 ·

JAIME RETAMALES

Retamales volunteered as legal assistant and teacher in an immigrant shelter and high security center in Texas. He taught Jeremias for 6 months in 2015. When Jeremias attempted to cross the U.S. border, he was caught by the border patrol. He was first sent to the detention center for adults and then to a facility for unaccompanied children. Jeremias always remembered his country and imagined himself freely walking the streets, enjoying the beach and the parks. His experience in the United States was inside of the walls of the detention center, and walls he saw every day. Unfortunately, one of his creative talents became his condemnation.

Jeremías

Jeremías es un muchacho hondureño, según la lista de clientes es un adolescente de dieciséis años, aunque, parece tener unos veinte. Seguramente, debió madurar temprano para ayudar a su familia como la mayoría de los niños que atendemos en este centro. Al igual que muchos habitantes de Honduras, en sus venas corre sangre africana que se hace evidente en su aspecto físico. Hace dos años que enseño en este lugar, todos los días llegan niños como Jeremías a los Estados Unidos con la esperanza de trabajar y enviar dinero para que sus madres no se maten buscando alimentos para sus hermanas o hermanos.

A Jeremías lo agarraron hace un mes, se entregó a la migra porque estaba perdido, sin agua, el coyote lo abandonó junto con el grupo en que venía después de oír al helicóptero de la patrulla fronteriza sobrevolar el lugar. Jeremías les dijo a los oficiales que era mayor de edad siguiendo el consejo del coyote, por eso lo mandaron a una cárcel con otros adultos, donde no lo pasó bien. Los mismos agentes se dieron cuenta que todavía era un niño y después de tres semanas lo mandaron a nuestro centro. Probablemente fue lo mejor, pues, no he escuchado nada bueno de esos lugares. Aquí puede vivir como un niño, pues si se porta bien, puede jugar fútbol con los otros muchachos, ver televisión, aprender manualidades y asistir a mis clases.

Llegó hace una semana, como los demás tímidamente se empezó a integrar a los otros cuarenta, que viven en forma provisional en este lugar. Jenny, su asistente social, en nuestra reunión semanal, me confesó que es difícil encontrar a un familiar para mandárselo, pues, son ellos también indocumentados y no quieren correr riesgos con Immigration and Customs Enforcement (ICE). Jeremías apenas sabe leer y escribir, y menos sabe de matemáticas, historia o ciencias. No me sorprende, la mayoría de los niños que llegan a este centro, apenas han cursado primaria. Desde niños han tenido que trabajar para ayudar a mantener a sus hermanos y hermanas. Jeremías quiere aprender, le pone empeño al estudio. Me dijo que estudiar le ayuda a distraerse, pues, cada día que pasa es un día sin mandar dinero a Honduras para ayudar a su madre. Sin darse cuenta ha aprendido las operaciones básicas de matemáticas, palabras en inglés, algo de historia y a dibujar. Me he dado de cuenta que es un artista, probablemente nadie se lo dijo, él no se lo cree, piensa que le miento cuando lo felicito por sus pinturas. No es la primera vez que tengo entre mis alumnos a uno que tiene un talento escondido. Ellos tienen prioridades como trabajar para conseguir alimentos, deben dejar de lado los estudios o la diversión.

Ya ha pasado un mes y nada. No hay familiar que quiera sacarlo, nada. El tiempo ha hecho mella en su personalidad, está más callado, absorto en sus pensamientos. Se le nota preocupado, deprimido, sabe que si no encuentran algún familiar tendrá que volver a su país. Le pregunto cómo está, me responde que bien, nada más, Pero, sus dibujos se han tornado más oscuros, turbios, los colores brillantes han variado a tonos opacos. Aunque siguen siendo hermosos. Las paredes de casi todas las oficinas tienen uno de ellos. Fue uno de sus trabajos que lo condenó. Inocentemente le dibujó a uno de sus amigos un Rambo, disparando y matando a sus enemigos. Jeremías me lo contó. El otro joven le daría unos dulces que guardaba en su gabinete. Uno de los empleados lo vio dibujándolo en el taller de pintura y lo acusó de planear un ataque. El director del centro vio una amenaza en contra de los empleados y los clientes, pues, el dibujo parecía una amenaza de venganza. Le pusieron dos guardianes que lo seguían a todas partes, le impidieron salir a jugar fútbol, a paseos, ver películas con otros clientes, le quitaron los lápices e iniciaron un protocolo de cambio a un centro de máxima seguridad. Aunque, varios empleados intercedimos por él, la suerte estaba echada. Jeremías, se dio cuenta que, si lo mandaban al centro de máxima seguridad, pasaría mucho tiempo detenido con muchachos violentos, miembros de pandillas o delincuentes juveniles. Habló con la asistente social, le dijo que no dibujaría más y que quería volver a su país. Lamentablemente, no basta con que lo diga, sino que tiene que comprobarlo.

El lunes llegué a trabajar y ya se habían llevado a Jeremías al centro de máxima seguridad. Vi sus dibujos pegados en las paredes de mi sala de clase. Eran doce, muy buenos, todos paisajes de su país, cabañas pobres de pescadores garífunas, todos se veían felices, algunos bailando o tocando instrumentos. También dibujó a su familia, numerosa, con la figura de la madre, no del padre, pero todos sonriendo. Me llamó la atención el único dibujo que hizo sobre los Estados Unidos, estaba lleno de muros y rejas, el único paisaje del país que había conocido hasta ahora.

Jeremías
Tara Marshall (Translator)

Jeremías is a Honduran boy, and according to the list of children, he is 16 years old but looks like he is twenty. Surely, he has matured early to help his family like the majority of the kids living at this center. Similar to many of the Honduran inhabitants, African blood runs in his veins and it shows in his physical appearance. I have been teaching in this place for 2 years now, and everyday children like Jeremías come to the United States with the hope of working and sending money so that their mothers do not kill themselves searching for nourishment for their brothers and sisters.

Jeremías was seized a month ago. He handed himself over to immigration officers because he was lost and without any water. The coyote abandoned him along with the rest of group when he heard the helicopter of the border patrol hovering over them. Jeremías told the officials that he was 18 years old, surely following the coyote's advice, and because of this they sent him to jail with other adults, where things did not go well. Agents realized that he was still a boy, and 3 weeks later, sent him to our center. It was probably for the best, well, I have not heard anything good about those places. Here he will be able to live as a child, if he behaves, play soccer with the other boys, watch television, make arts and crafts, and attend my classes.

He arrived a week ago, like the others he began to integrate timidly with the forty other children who live provisionally in this place. In our weekly meeting, Jenny, our social worker, confessed to me that it is difficult to find a family member for him because they also are undocumented and don't want to run risks with Immigration and Customs Enforcement (ICE). Jeremías can hardly read or write, and knows little of math, history, or science. It doesn't surprise me; the majority of children who come to this center have barely attended primary school because they had to work to support their brothers and sisters. Jeremías wants to learn; he pays attention to his studies. He told me that studying helps distract him from the fact that each day that passes is a day that he can't send money back to Honduras for his mother. Without realizing it, he has already learned basic mathematical operations, words in English, some history, and how to draw. I noticed that he is a good artist, though probably no one has told him, and he certainly doesn't believe it; he thinks that I'm lying whenever I congratulate him about his drawings. This isn't the first time I have had someone with a hidden talent amongst my students. They had priorities like working to provide food, so they had to put aside their talents, studies, and fun.

A month has already passed and nothing. There is not a relative that wants to take him at all. Time has taken its toll on his spirit: he is quieter, absorbed in his thoughts. He is worried, depressed, for he knows that if they do not find a family member he will have to return to his country. When I ask him how he is feeling, he responds, "good," and nothing more. But his drawings have turned darker, turbulent; the vibrant colors have gone opaque, although they are still beautiful. Almost all of our offices have one of his drawings on the wall. One of them condemned him, though. Innocently, he drew one of his friends as Rambo, shooting and killing his enemies. Jeremías told me that he painted it because the other young man would give him some sweets that he kept in his cabinet. One of the employees saw him drawing this piece in the art room and accused him of planning an attack. The center's director viewed it as a threat against the employees and clients because the drawing could be interpreted as if Jeremias was depicting revenge. They put two guards in charge, who would follow him everywhere, they prevented him from playing soccer, walking, or seeing movies with the other clients. They took his pencils. A protocol to change him to a maximum-security center started. Although several employees interceded on his behalf, his fate was already decided. Jeremías, realized that if he was sent to the center, he would spend a lot of time with violent boys, gang members and juvenile delinquents. He spoke with the social worker saying he would never draw again and that he wanted to return to his country. Unfortunately, it was not enough; he had to prove it.

Monday when I arrived at work, they had already taken Jeremías to the maximum-security shelter. I saw his drawings pinned on the walls of my classroom. There were twelve excellent landscapes of his country, poor huts of Garífuna fishermen, all looking very happy, some dancing or playing instruments. He also drew his numerous family members and his mother, but not his father. All of them were smiling. I was struck by the only drawing he made of the United States; it was full of walls and bars, the only landscape in the country he had known so far here.

Part IV

THE LOVE OF STRANGERS

LUZ M. GARCINI AND
MARTIN LA ROCHE

Garcini and La Roche write the account of their recent relationship with Juan, an undocumented 18-year old adolescent at the hospice in California where they provided him with palliative care in 2014. A native of a small rural town in Northern Mexico, Juan was born with a congenital heart defect and according to his physicians his life expectancy was no more than 15 years. Given his mother's lack of financial resources and inadequate access to medical care, Juan's chances for survival in Mexico were slim. Thus, his mother, determined to give her son a chance to live, embarked him on a journey to the United States. Her hope was to find a new heart for Juan that would save his life

An Undocumented Journey in Search of a Heart[1]

I first met Juan, a thin 18-year-old who smiled with his eyes, at the inpatient hospice unit where I worked (first author). His mother, Guadalupe, sat beside him as he struggled to breathe. Despite his difficulties, he cheerfully looked directly into my eyes and said in Spanish "*Hola Doctora*, do you want to hear my favorite Bible verse? 'I will give you a new heart, and I will put a new spirit within you', *Ezequiel* 36:26." He then kept silent for a few seconds perhaps battling with the dose of morphine that he had just received. He added, "I never got a new heart, but I kept the spirit." Juan was born with a congenital heart defect and, according to his physicians, his life expectancy was no more than 15 years. Given Guadalupe's lack of financial resources and inadequate access to medical care, Juan's chances for survival in the small rural town of Alamos in Northern Mexico were slim. Guadalupe became a widow at the age of twenty after Juan's father died in a work-related accident at a copper mine; she had both limited education and a lacking support system. Her family had chastised her after she became pregnant with Juan, and she often found herself taking care of him alone. Regardless, she was a woman of courage, and she was determined to give her son a chance to live. She embarked on a journey to the United States with the hope that she would find a new heart for Juan.

When I met Juan, he had been admitted to the hospice 3 weeks before. The hospice provides holistic, palliative care to chronically and terminally ill patients when clinical care is no longer sufficient to manage the patient's pain and symptoms. Most commonly, it is a place aimed at providing a peaceful death while attending to the physical, emotional, and spiritual needs of patients and their families. The hospice would be the last setting—out of many—in which Juan would be held. Many other detention settings had left profound psychological wounds. For instance, not too long ago, he was taken to an immigration detention center upon being victim of a raid at a Mexican restaurant while having dinner with members of his church. This event was so distressing for him that, shortly after his arrival to the detention center, Juan collapsed and had to be released due to medical need and taken to the hospital's intensive care unit. Since that arrest, Juan's health rapidly declined. Guadalupe explained that she believed that this event was so traumatic that it killed Juan's heart. However, she asserted that his spirit remains strong.

Despite the many adversities that Juan had faced, he not only found strength to support himself, but also his mother. He paid as much attention to her needs as she did to his. At times, they seemed to complete their sentences and other times they would seem to speak volumes by just looking at each other. Both Juan and Guadalupe seemed to have a connection that was bigger than the sum of each one alone. It was a mutual understanding based on love, but also on something more. Perhaps, it was because both of them shared a similar experience. They both awaited death while also witnessing the gradual loss of the person that they loved most. Four years before, Guadalupe was diagnosed with autoimmune hepatitis. Her disease progressed so rapidly that only a liver transplant would have saved her life. Like Juan, her chances for a transplant were slim given her undocumented status and limited financial resources.

Nevertheless, despite the many difficult times that Juan and Guadalupe had faced, they were always open and even thankful for my words and efforts to be with them. Often, after I left the room, my heart was beating more strongly, and I was thankful for the opportunity to have met them. Juan and Guadalupe were equally well liked by the nurses and doctors in the unit, who also enjoyed spending time with them. Some of them would say that Juan's resilience and love for his mother was remarkable, and a nurse even described him as "the eye in a storm, where peace can be found." Likewise, they described Guadalupe as an exemplary mother whose priority was her son and who was always grateful for the care provided.

The hospice is the final destination for many different people; however, few were as young as Juan. It is difficult to think of the many chapters in Juan's life that he will not get to live. Since his arrival at the unit, I visited him often and although the effects of sedation often got in the way of our conversations, I learned about his experiences and frustrations, sometimes through his own words, sometimes through Guadalupe's. Juan described how it wasn't until the age of ten that he and his mother gave up their hope for a heart transplant upon hearing from doctors that it was already too late for this option and that there was not much else to be done. The years prior to that were spent frantically trying to gain access to medical treatment, which was limited due to financial strain and his undocumented status. The last 8 years were spent aiming for access to clinical trials, including stem cell transplants, that would buy Juan more time. But, once again, it was too late even for those options. As I walked into his dimly lit room, I was often reminded that for him, "to live" means to be hooked up to an oxygen tank that facilitates his breathing and depend on high doses of morphine to avoid the pain.

I had first learned about Juan from a chart review. In the demographic section, it read "charity care," which often hints at the patient's undocumented status. Determined to meet my goal as a provider, that is, "to help patients cope with loss and celebrate life as the end comes near," I looked for a time that I could talk to Juan to gain better insight into his history—when the effects of morphine wouldn't interfere too much with our conversation. Growing up with a heart defect had been painful. Juan had often experienced fatigue, pulmonary hypertension, a persistent cough, shortness of breath, painful swelling, chest pain, purple bruising, dizziness, and severe fatigue. However, at times it was even more difficult for him to cope with the stress of being undocumented. He often feared that he and his mother would be deported. Many times, he felt marginalized and discriminated against because of their status. Juan often felt he had been rendered voiceless, invisible, and treated as if he was a criminal. Even during his sleep, he would often be trapped in endless nightmares about being detained and separated from his mother. However, after waking up, his reality seemed as unfair and harsh as his nightmares.

He once told me, after singing the words of a Mexican song, "*no soy de aquí, ni soy de allá* [I am not from here, nor from there]," that he struggled to develop a sense of belonging since he lived in between two cultures, neither of which he considered his own and neither of which accepted him. On one hand, he had lived in the United States for most of his life. He felt unwanted in the country in which he grew up and was often treated as an undeserving boy or criminal. On the other hand, he knew very little about life in Mexico; so little that it was hard for him to claim roots to his native country. Despite struggling with a sense of belonging, Juan knew only one way to live: to keep having faith in the midst of disadvantage, uncertainty, and adversity. He planned his life as if the end was not near and everyday was a gift. For instance, he had worked hard to become a stellar student so that he could defy existing stereotypes that Mexicans are lazy and so that his mother would feel proud of him. He had also been a devoted member of his church and volunteered at their youth groups so that he could make others like himself feel *en familia*. He had helped his mother sell *tamales* to make ends meet. For him, making each *tamal* was like making a piece of art. He would pour all his heart into the *tamal* hoping that it would be better than the previous one.

It was also from a chart review that I first learned about Juan's psychosocial challenges... a long list of the different mental health disorders for which he met criteria read "recurrent major depressive disorder, lifetime panic attacks, generalized anxiety disorder, post-traumatic stress disorder, and drug dependence (morphine)." I realized that although Juan had never had a drink of alcohol or used recreational drugs, he was described as suffering from a drug dependent disorder. If included within an epidemiological study, he would be another data point indicating an undocumented immigrant who is a drug addict. I wondered about how many more faceless numbers and stories of injustice are buried under a diagnostic category.

Guadalupe had once commented that Juan was attracted to men and that he was very confused and anxious about these feelings. Furthermore, Juan did not talk much about these issues because he feared that people might blame his mother for raising him gay and without a father figure. Guadalupe was also feeling confused because she did not know how to help him or guide him. She had often heard others criticize gay men for not being *macho*. However, Guadalupe knew this was not the case and she tried to help her son open up and talk about these and other issues.

As providers, we often rely on chart reviews to learn the most important details about our patient's stories. However, there is no section in a chart that lists a patient's dreams, which can often tell us much more about a person than a diagnostic label or a demographic profile. Juan's dream was to become a "heart doctor" so that he could help others like himself. One day, upon asking him why he wanted to be a doctor, he said, *adonde el corazón camina, el pie se inclina* [where the heart walks, the foot follows]. Juan had more life hardship than most children of his age, and he did not want others to go through the pain that he had suffered. Another of Juan's dreams was to have a large traditional family that would stay together and would help others cope with their immigration status problems. "Life is an opportunity to give and enrich others," he would repeat. He enjoyed welcoming me with a Bible verse from the many that he had memorized. I would never forget the day he taught me about "the fruits of the spirit" from the book of Galatians. He said, "*Doctora*, do you know that there is no law against love, joy, peace, patience, kindness, goodness, faithfulness, gentleness and self-control. . . the world would be a better place if we could practice this a bit more." As I heard him speak while looking at the blue tint of his skin, I was deeply moved, and my eyes welled up. I wondered if I would see him again. Would he have another day to live?

I feared that Juan's hopes would fade and be forgotten. Even now, as we write Juan's story, we feel our hearts pound quickly. However, our hearts beat more strongly and confidently because we have been touched by his heart, a heart filled with love, tolerance, and compassion. As we write these paragraphs, we hope that some of what we have received from Juan touches you and helps us go beyond walls and borders. Many of these walls are not only being built along our southern border but are also cultural categories that divide us according to skin color, socioeconomic status, or place of birth. In a time in which so many are being forgotten or stigmatized, it is important to listen and acknowledge each and all of us. Although Juan never got his heart from America, he nevertheless gave us so much more, particularly to the two authors of this story. Our mission is renewed; we feel ready and reenergized to listen and acknowledge others, regardless their skin color, gender orientation, religious background or documentation status. Our hearts are reinvigorated because of Juan.

Un viaje indocumentado en busca de un corazón[2]

Mercedes Fernández Asenjo (Translator)

La primera vez que conocí a Juan, un muchacho delgado de 18 años, con una sonrisa en su mirada, estaba en una clínica de corta estancia donde yo trabajaba (primer autor). Su madre, Guadalupe, estaba sentada cerca de él porque le costaba respirar. A pesar de sus dificultades, Juan me miró directamente a los ojos y dijo de manera muy alegre "*Hola Doctora*, ¿quiere escuchar mi versículo preferido de la Biblia? 'Te daré un corazón nuevo y pondré un nuevo espíritu dentro de ti,' *Ezequiel* 36:26". Luego permaneció en silencio durante unos segundos mientras combatía contra la dosis de morfina que acababa de recibir. Añadió, "Nunca recibí un corazón nuevo, pero mantengo las esperanzas." Juan había nacido con un defecto congénito en el corazón y, según las previsiones de sus médicos, su esperanza de vida no superaría los quince años. Debido a la falta de recursos financieros de Guadalupe y al deficiente acceso a un buen cuidado médico, las posibilidades de que Juan sobreviviera en el pequeño pueblo rural de los Álamos en el norte de México eran mínimas. Guadalupe había enviudado a los veinte años después del fallecimiento del padre de Juan en un accidente laboral en la mina de cobre donde trabajaba. Su familia le dio la espalda cuando supieron que estaba embarazada y en repetidas ocasiones se encontró a sí misma haciéndose cargo del bebé ella sola. A pesar de todas las adversidades, era una mujer fuerte y estaba decidida a darle a su hijo la oportunidad de vivir. Se embarcó en un viaje hacia los Estados Unidos con la esperanza de encontrar un nuevo corazón para Juan.

Cuando conocí a Juan, lo habían admitido en el hospital para enfermos terminales tres semanas antes. Este lugar ofrece cuidados paliativos y holísticos para pacientes crónicos y terminales cuando el tratamiento clínico ya no es suficiente para paliar el dolor y los síntomas de estos pacientes. Por lo general es un lugar diseñado para proporcionarles una muerte tranquila mientras se atiende a sus necesidades físicas, emocionales y espirituales y a las de sus familias. Este hospital sería el último de otros muchos en el que Juan estuvo detenido. Otros centros de detención le habían dejado profundas heridas psicológicas. Por ejemplo, poco tiempo atrás, lo llevaron a un centro de detención tras una redada en un restaurante mexicano donde estaba cenando con otros miembros de su iglesia. Este hecho fue tan inquietante para él que, al poco tiempo de llegar al centro de detención, Juan sufrió un colapso nervioso y lo tuvieron que poner en libertad a causa de una exigencia médica y mandarlo a la unidad de cuidados intensivos del hospital. Desde aquel arresto, la salud de Juan empeoró rápidamente. Guadalupe me explicó que ella estaba convencida de que este hecho fue tan traumático para su hijo que acabó con su corazón. Aun así, ella creía que su ánimo permanecía fuerte.

A pesar de la gran cantidad de adversidades a las que Juan se había enfrentado, no sólo encontró la fuerza para sobrellevarlas, sino también para que su madre lo hiciera, prestando tanta atención a las necesidades de ella como a las suyas. A veces, parecía que se completaban las frases mientras que en otras circunstancias parecía que se decían mucho sólo mirándose el uno al otro. Era como si los dos tuvieran una conexión más grande que la suma de cada uno por separado. Se trataba de un entendimiento mutuo basado en el amor, pero también en algo más. Quizás era porque ambos compartían una experiencia similar, ya que los dos estaban esperando morirse mientras presenciaban la pérdida gradual de la persona que más querían. Cuatro años antes, a Guadalupe le habían diagnosticado una hepatitis autoinmune. Su enfermedad avanzó tan rápidamente que sólo un trasplante de hígado le hubiera salvado la vida, pero como a Juan, las posibilidades de que se lo hicieran eran mínimas debido a su estatus de indocumentada y a sus limitados recursos financieros.

Sin embargo, a pesar de todos los momentos difíciles que Juan y Guadalupe habían afrontado, siempre estaban abiertos e incluso agradecidos por mis palabras y por mis esfuerzos para pasar tiempo con ellos. Con frecuencia, después de salir de su habitación, mi corazón latía con más intensidad y yo agradecía la oportunidad de haberlos conocido. Los doctores y las enfermeras de la unidad de cuidados paliativos querían por igual a Juan y a Guadalupe, y también disfrutaban cuando pasaban tiempo con ellos. Algunos decían que la resiliencia de Juan y el amor hacia su madre eran extraordinarios, y una enfermera incluso describía a Juan como "el ojo de la tormenta donde se encuentra la paz". De la misma manera, describían a Guadalupe como una madre ejemplar cuya prioridad era su hijo y que siempre mostraba su gratitud por los cuidados que se le proporcionaban.

El hospital para enfermos terminales es el destino final para mucha gente diferente; pero pocos eran tan jóvenes como Juan. Es difícil pensar cuántas cosas Juan no llegaría a vivir. Desde su llegada a la unidad de cuidados intensivos, lo visitaba con frecuencia y aunque los efectos de la sedación a menudo interrumpían nuestras conversaciones, logré conocer sus experiencias y sus frustraciones; a veces a través de sus propias palabras, otras, por las de Guadalupe. Juan me describió cómo, al cumplir diez años, su madre y él abandonaron la esperanza de que le hicieran un trasplante de corazón cuando los doctores les comunicaron que ya era demasiado tarde para intentar esta opción y que ya había poco que hacer. Los años anteriores a esa noticia los pasaron frenéticamente intentando conseguir acceso a un tratamiento médico que era limitado a causa de sus escasos recursos económicos y de su condición de indocumentados. Los últimos ocho años intentaron por todos los medios acceder a pruebas clínicas experimentales, entre ellas trasplantes de células madre, que le habrían permitido a Juan ampliar su esperanza de vida. Pero, una vez más, era demasiado tarde incluso para esas opciones. Cuando caminaba hacia su habitación tenuemente iluminada, a menudo me recordaba a mí misma que para él "vivir" significaba estar enchufado a un tanque de oxígeno que le facilitaba respirar y que dependía de altas dosis de morfina para evitarle el dolor.

La primera vez que supe acerca de Juan fue mientras revisaba una gráfica. En la sección demográfica, se apuntaba "cuidado suministrado por los servicios de caridad/ cuidado de caridad", lo que a menudo es una pista sobre el estatus de indocumentado del paciente. Determinada a cumplir con mi objetivo de proveedora [de servicios médicos], es decir, "de ayudar a los pacientes a superar la pérdida y a celebrar la vida mientras ésta llega a su fin," busqué un momento en el que pudiese hablar con Juan, cuando los efectos de la morfina no interfirieran demasiado en nuestra conversación, para lograr comprender mejor su historia. El hecho de crecer con un defecto en el corazón había sido doloroso ya que, a menudo, Juan experimentaba fatiga, hipertensión pulmonar, tos persistente, insuficiencia respiratoria, tumefacción dolorosa, dolor de pecho, moratones, mareo y fatiga extrema. Sin embargo, a veces era incluso más difícil para él lidiar con el estrés de ser indocumentado. Con frecuencia temía que los deportaran a su madre y a él. En muchas ocasiones, se sintió marginado y discriminado a causa de su estatus. Incluso durante el sueño, frecuentemente se veía a sí mismo atrapado en pesadillas sin fin en las que lo detenían y lo separaban de su madre. Al despertarse, de todos modos, la realidad circunstante le parecía tan injusta y hostil como la de sus pesadillas.

Una vez me dijo, después de cantar la letra de una canción mexicana que decía "no soy de aquí, ni soy de allá", que a él le costaba trabajo desarrollar un sentimiento de pertenencia puesto que había vivido entre dos culturas a las que no consideraba suyas y que ninguna de las dos lo había aceptado. Por una parte, había transcurrido la mayor parte de su vida en los Estados Unidos, pero no se sentía querido en el país donde había crecido porque a menudo lo trataban como si fuera un niño indigno o un criminal. Por otro lado, sabía muy poco de su vida en México, tan poco que le era difícil reivindicar sus raíces al país que lo vio nacer. A pesar de luchar con este sentido de pertenencia, Juan sólo conocía una forma de vivir, que consistía en mantener sus creencias en medio de la desventaja, la incerteza y la adversidad. Planeaba su vida como si el final no estuviera cerca y como si cada día fuese un regalo. Por ejemplo, había trabajado muy duro para convertirse en un estudiante estrella y desafiar así el estereotipo de que los mexicanos son holgazanes y hacer que su madre se sintiera orgullosa de él. También había sido un miembro devoto de su congregación y había sido voluntario con los grupos juveniles con el objetivo de hacer que otros muchachos como él se sintieran "en familia." Había ayudado a su madre a vender tamales para poder llegar a finales de mes. Para él, preparar cada *tamal* era como hacer una obra de arte, y ponía todo su corazón en cada nuevo tamal con la esperanza de que fuese mejor que el anterior.

Fue también después de revisar una gráfica cuando me enteré por primera vez de los desafíos psicosociales de Juan ... una larga lista de diferentes desórdenes mentales que entraban en la categoría de "trastorno depresivo mayor recurrente, ataques de pánico de por vida, trastorno de ansiedad generalizado, trastorno de estrés post-traumático y dependencia a la morfina." Me di cuenta de que a pesar de que Juan nunca había bebido alcohol o usado drogas, se le describía como si sufriese un trastorno derivado del consumo habitual de drogas. Si lo hubieran incluido dentro de un estudio epidemiológico, representaría un dato más, e indicaría que se trataba de un inmigrante indocumentado y drogadicto. Me preguntaba entonces cuántos casos más sin rostro e historias injustas están enterrados bajo una categoría diagnóstica.

Guadalupe había comentado una vez que a Juan le atraían los hombres y que se sentía muy confundido y preocupado frente a estos sentimientos. Además, Juan no hablaba mucho sobre ello porque temía que la gente acusara a su madre de haberlo educado como un homosexual y sin una figura paterna. Guadalupe también se sentía confundida porque no sabía cómo ayudarlo u orientarlo. Con frecuencia había escuchado a otras personas criticar a los homosexuales por no ser *machos*. Sin embargo, ella sabía que éste no era el caso de Juan e intentaba ayudar a que su hijo se sincerara y hablase de éste y de otros temas.

Como proveedores [de servicios médicos], a menudo confiamos en los datos de las gráficas para saber los detalles más relevantes del historial médico de nuestros pacientes. Pero no existe una sección dentro de la gráfica que enumere los sueños del paciente. Juan soñaba con convertirse en un "doctor del corazón" para poder ayudar a otros como él. Un día, al preguntarle el porqué de este deseo, me dijo "adonde el corazón camina, el pie se inclina." Juan había sufrido más adversidades en su vida que el resto de los niños de su edad, y no quería que otros tuvieran que pasar por el dolor que él había experimentado. Otro de sus sueños era tener una gran familia tradicional que estuviera unida y que se ayudase a sobrellevar los problemas derivados de su condición migratoria. "La vida es una oportunidad de dar y enriquecer a otros," solía repetir. Disfrutaba dándome la bienvenida con un verso de la Biblia de los muchos que se sabía de memoria. Nunca olvidaré el día que me enseñó acerca de "los frutos del espíritu" del libro de los Gálatas. Me dijo, "Doctora, ¿sabe que no hay una ley en contra del amor, la felicidad, la paz, la paciencia, la bondad, la generosidad, la lealtad, la gentileza y el autocontrol . . . ? El mundo sería un lugar mejor si todos comulgáramos con esto un poquito más." Me conmoví cuando lo escuché hablar mientras se miraba el tono azulado de su piel, y mis ojos se llenaron de lágrimas. Me pregunté si lo volvería a ver de nuevo y si él tendría un día más de vida.

Temía que las esperanzas de Juan desaparecieran y cayeran en el olvido. Incluso ahora, cuando escribimos la historia de Juan, sentimos que nuestros corazones laten con fuerza. Sin embargo, nuestros corazones palpitan de manera más fuerte y con más seguridad porque todos nosotros nos conmovimos con el suyo, un corazón rebosante de amor, tolerancia y compasión. Al escribir estos párrafos, esperamos que algo de lo que nosotros recibimos de Juan les llegue y nos permita ir más allá de los muros y de las fronteras. Muchos de estos muros no se construyen sólo a lo largo de nuestra frontera sur, sino que son categorías culturales que nos dividen según el color de piel, el estatus socioeconómico, o el lugar de nacimiento. En un momento en el que muchos seres humanos están siendo olvidados o estigmatizados, es importante escuchar y aceptarnos los unos a los otros. Aunque Juan nunca consiguió su corazón en América, él nos dio mucho más, especialmente a los dos autores de este relato. Se renovó nuestra misión; nos sentimos listos y llenos de energía para escuchar y aceptar a otras personas sin importarnos su color de piel, su orientación sexual, sus creencias religiosas o el estatus migratorio. Nuestros corazones están renovados gracias a Juan.

Notes

1. Disclosures: The authors of this manuscript have no conflict of interests to disclose. Acknowledgment: Funding was provided to Luz Garcini by the Ford Fellowship.
2. Declaración de confidencialidad: Los autores de este manuscrito no tienen conflicto de intereses para su divulgación. Agradecimientos: La Beca Ford proporcionó la financiación a Luz Garcini para este proyecto.

· 1 2 ·

JUAN A. RÍOS VEGA

Ríos Vega reflects on his teaching journey teaching undocumented immigrant students, 16 to 18 years of age, in a middle and high school in the Southeast from 1999 to 2012. Student dialogue journals and Ríos Vega's testimony are two forms of data collection in a qualitative study that claims his classroom was a healing place by the sharing their similar experiences of oppression and marginalization they suffered as newcomers.

An ESL Classroom as a Healing Space

I carry my students' journals with me as personal treasures. Wherever I go, I try to share them with future student teachers so they can learn from my former English as a Second Language (ESL) students' personal narratives. I promised myself to share my former students' narratives with others. I always wanted more individuals to learn what it means to be a Latinx immigrant tee-nager in the United States. In this essay, I share the written narratives of three of my former ESL students, Sheila, William, and Carlos. Amazingly, what started as a classroom writing project over 10 years ago, where students were encouraged to write about their personal stories, turned into biographical arti-facts in narrative research,[1] to echo the personal experiences Latinx youth in education. These three narratives explore issues of immigration journeys, *familia*, discrimination, and racism. Unfortunately, two of the students in this paper, Sheila and William, passed away a couple of years ago.

Carlos's narrative of gender discrimination and xenophobia allowed me to better understand the inner world of many Latinx youth and their families in this country, especially those who do not speak the dominant language and those who always fear of being deported for not having their legal immigration papers. These three Latinx students, as well as many others, have given me the strength and empowerment to write this piece.

When I came to the U.S. as an exchange teacher from my beloved Panama over 20 years ago, I assumed that I was going to teach English-speaking students to speak Spanish, as some of my friends told me before I moved here. However, to my surprise, my students were English language learners (ELLs) from Mexico, Guatemala, El Salvador, Nicaragua, Honduras, Costa Rica, Panama, Dominican Republic, Puerto Rico, Colombia, and Venezuela, as well as Pakistan, India, Vietnam, and so many other countries around the globe.

I have to confess that moving to the Southeast U.S. was a culture shock for me. I learned that some social issues such as racism and xenophobia were still alive. I quickly learned that schools were racially segregated and that brown-skinned and Spanish-speaking people like myself were racially profiled as "illegal immigrants." Before coming to this country, I never spent time to question my skin color, my Spanish accent while speaking English, and my presence in certain spaces. After my arrival, there were times when I thought my skin color and "accent" did not qualify me as "smart." I sometimes felt invisible or unwelcomed by others, especially colleagues or locals. There were many instances when I wanted to go back to my country. I felt hurt and frustrated.

Once I started teaching, I discovered that my students and I shared many things in common besides being immigrants. We became a *familia* and the ESL classroom became our *hogar*—our healing space. There was not a single day when I did not learn something from my students and their families. Many of my students were not aware that they empowered me to become not only a teacher in the classroom but a leader in the community, and a Latinx scholar.

At the beginning of my teaching experience, I found it difficult to get students engaged about learning the English language. I noticed students felt oppressed and marginalized, especially when other teachers and students would tell them, "Speak English, this is America" or "if you want to speak Spanish, go back to Mexico."

After attending some conferences, I learned about the importance of using culturally relevant curriculum in the classroom. I immediately fell in love with Latinx authors like Sandra Cisneros, Pat Mora, Isabel Allende, Francisco Jiménez, Gary Soto, and Julia Alvarez. Their books allowed me and my students to find common ground to unpack and to critically analyze our personal experiences as immigrants. Together, we discovered that we were not alone. Instead, our reading experiences led us to talk about family and gender expectations, gangs, love, drugs, teen pregnancy, poverty, and hopes. We were also able to learn how other immigrants and Latinx people faced the same social problems that my students and I experienced on a daily basis.

Reading about racism, classism, immigration, English language learning, and schooling through the eyes of the authors' characters served as a springboard for my students to reflect and to write their own stories. In 2008, I decided to use Sandra Cisneros's famous book, *A House on Mango Street*, as an inspiration for my students to develop their personal narratives. After reading and learning about Esperanza and her Latino neighborhood in Chicago, I realized how important it was for my students to understand that their personal stories were also valuable and welcome in my classroom. Every day, after reading one or two vignettes from Cisneros's book, my students wrote about their lives in their personal journals. They wrote about their names, their neighborhoods back in their countries and in North Carolina, a birth in the family, their teachers, their immigration journeys, and experiences with feeling unwelcome in the new country.

After reading and prompting my students with more questions about their personal journals, I decided to turn it into a writing project. One day I showed them the film *Freedom Writers* because I wanted them to have an idea of what I wanted them to do with their narratives. After watching the film, Sheila, the student about whom I will talk later said, "That teacher is like you, Mr. Ríos." When I heard Sheila realize how much I cared about their personal stories, I felt a knot form in my throat, and I almost cried.

Once my students finished writing personal stories in their journals, I took the students to the school computer lab so they could type their stories. It was so powerful to witness my students' enthusiasm about becoming authors of their own books, as I called them. While they were typing, I walked around the room asking them to include more details about their stories.

When they finished typing and editing their stories, I taught them how to create a front cover and how to bind their books. They also included a dedication and a table of contents. Some others decided to include pictures and stickers, as well as their own drawings and titles. Once their books were finally finished, I organized a party to celebrate their books. We brought foods and drinks. During our celebration, I asked students to make a circle and to pick one of their stories to be read aloud. When they read their pieces, we all laughed, reflected, asked more questions, and also wept. I recall when Veronica, a Mexican student, wrote about me in her dedication. She cried and made me cry while sharing how thankful she was to have me as her teacher. That year Veronica turned 15. We surprised her with a cake and soft drinks since her mother could not afford to have a *quinceañera* party for her. Students like Veronica and so many others shaped my life as a human being and a teacher. I have kept my students' journals since then. I always thought about sharing their personal narratives with others.

Sheila came to the United States and started as a freshman in 2004. She always showed her happiness and willingness to learn the new language. She was very smart and talented. She loved to draw and to decorate things. Additionally, she was an excellent dancer and loved to participate in a Mexican folk-dance group that I also organized at school. After she moved back to Mexico with her family, we were still friends via Facebook for over 2 years. Sheila shared pictures of her wedding and crafts. She seemed to be very content back in her homeland. Unfortunately, on October 10, 2014, another student emailed me the bad news that Sheila had passed away after a heart surgery. It was devastating to accept Sheila's early departure. She will always be in my heart and my thoughts. This is Sheila's personal journal about her immigration journey when she was my student.

My Journey to the United States

Everything occurred so fast, just two months after my dad left us to come to the US, my mom decided to come with him. She sold everything, the car, clothes, furniture, everything we had. Finally, she rented the house, and, in that moment, I knew it was the time to leave Mexico and with it my life. Because everything passed so quickly, we didn't even have time to say goodbye to the people we loved. One day I woke up and my mom told me and my brother, "We are leaving today; we are going with your dad. We have to be together like the family we are."

That day we got on the bus to Nuevo Laredo. There a woman was waiting for us. She looked weird, but we had to go with her if we wanted to be with my dad again. She talked to my mom and then my mom said that everything she was doing was because of us, my brother and me, because she loves us, and we were the most important people in her life. At the beginning, I didn't know what was going on until she told me, "Sheila, I have to go other way. I'm going to cross through the river to the other side, but you're going with your brother, please mi'ja take care of him and yourself." I was so scared because I didn't want to let my mom go, but I didn't have any other choice. I had to be responsible and take care of my brother. Since that day, I became a woman. My mom trusted me, and I couldn't betray her. My mom hugged us and while crying she let us know how much she loved us. Then she left. We passed two days without my mom. Those were the hardest days for me and my brother, but they helped me to grow up. I wasn't anymore a little girl. I was the person not just protecting myself but protecting my brother's life.

The second night my brother and I were in Houston, Texas, at my Uncle's house waiting for news about my mom. They called my uncle to let him know that my mom was safe and that she was on her way to Houston. I was so happy when she got home. When she saw us, she started to cry and to kiss us. She told us that she will never leave us behind again. That was a promise. We spent some days in Houston, but then we took our way to North Carolina where my dad was waiting for us.

Sheila's immigration story was commonly shared by others in my classroom. Most of them left their grandparents, relatives, and friends behind to reunite with their parents, usually their fathers, who left their countries first, saved some money, and paid a *coyote* (human smuggler) to bring them to the United States. It was always heartbreaking to hear my students' stories about seeing their parents after many years. Some of them recalled hugging and kissing wrong men mistaken as their fathers; others confessed having a tough life living with their biological parents since they were used to their grandparents whom they recognized as their real parents.

One of the most eye-opening experiences that impacted my life the most was listening or reading my students' immigration journeys about crossing dangerous rivers and borders. I read *testimonios* of young girls dressed as boys to avoid being raped by *coyotes*, children dressed in black garments or naked to avoid being seen by immigration officials, crossing the border with fake passports, and seeing people dying. I also read stories of poverty, hunger, single mothers, murdered parents and relatives, older siblings left behind, or the funeral of a grandparent or other relative that they could not attend. Moreover, I also read stories of hope and pride, especially when my students talked about their parents and how appreciative they were of the sacrifices they made to come to the United States. Students like William wanted to do well in school as a way to pay his mother back for all of her efforts to give him a better life.

William was a handsome Mexican teenager. He was always in love. He enjoyed dressing up nicely. He was very respectful and full of energy. Like some Latinx teenage boys, he also got into trouble while hanging out with the wrong people. I used to advise him a lot about life choices, girlfriends, and family. His mother and I became good friends, and she knew how much I cared about her son. I called her when he got into trouble in school, and she called me when he had broken the law in the community. William's journey in this world was very short. He was only 23 when he died in a car accident on November 28, 2015. I was in shock when I received the news on my cell phone. I was on my way to visit one of my former students and I let her know about William's tragedy. When I attended William's visitation, I gave my condolences to his mother. It broke my heart into pieces to witness such a tragic scene. By the time William died, he was the father of a 2-year-boy with his high school sweetheart. It had never crossed my mind that one of my closest students would die so soon. I felt I was having a bad dream when I saw William's dead body lying on that metal platform in a red plaid shirt, blue jeans, and a Mexican sombrero. I cannot erase that scene of a mother mourning her son's death.

William loved his mother and younger sister so much. He always talked very highly about his hardworking mother and his goal to become an architect back in Mexico. This is what he wrote in his personal journal in 2008:

Dear Mr. Ríos,

My name is William Hernandez. I am fifteen years old. I live in the town of Asheboro, North Carolina. I have black hair and brown skin. I am an honest person who likes to respect other people and help others. I like to write and to play soccer.

During the week, I go to school in the mornings. When I return home, first, I help my mom with the house chores and then I eat. I live with my mom and my sister. We help each other. When I finish helping my mom, sometimes I do my homework and listen to music. Since my dad doesn't live with us, we live in a small apartment.

Now, my mother has a boyfriend, who wants to marry her and take us to Charlotte, so we could have a better life. My mother is a hardworking and honest woman. She helps me a lot. I love her so much. My sister is six years old. She goes to kindergarten. I love her so much because she is cool. Well, sometimes she is mean because she took my place and now every person says that she is cute and everything, so I'm not the cute one anymore. Anyways, I'm proud to have such a family.

That is all I can say about me and my lovely family.

Dear Mr. Ríos,

My mom's name is Belen, and she is thirty-six years old. She is a hardworking mother. She likes to help older people, so people can help her back. What I like the most about my mom is that she gets mad about everything. She is an honest person. She works at a factory, but her salary is not too much, so she has to work a lot just for her children. She loves us so much, and everything she wants is a better life for us. She likes to dress up in a very nice looking way not to show off to others. She does it because that's the way she is, and she is so pretty.

The only thing my mom wants is to be happy. She wants to marry her boyfriend Alberto, because he is a nice person. He loves my mom and takes care of us, but especially my sister. My mom wants the best and I think she will be proud if I finish high school and graduate.

My mom got here about six or seven years ago. Since then, she has worked to save money and to send it to México to build a house and to have a place where we can live a better life.

William graduated from high school and continued working in a furniture factory with other young Latinx peers. Unfortunately, he split with his son's mother and started dating another girl. Like William, many Latinx youth realized that their dreams of pursuing higher education was an impossible task due to their immigration status. As a result, most undocumented Latinx end up working in factories, fast food restaurants, construction, and landscaping. Others decide to drop out of school due to a lack of a supportive system that can help them cope with low expectations of society and school. It always concerned me when I was told that a student decided to stop coming to school. Sometimes my students used to tell me lies about their decisions to drop out of school since they knew how much I disliked the idea. I used to instill in them that it was their time to remain in school and to get their high school diploma. I used my own example of staying focused with their life goals. I shared my story about pursuing graduate school in this country and how many years I patiently waited to be considered as an in-state tuition student. Some of them listened to my *consejos* (advice) while others, like Carlos, had a hard time keeping up with society and life's obstacles.

Carlos was the son I always wanted to have. He reminded me so much of my older brother. When he came to my high school, he had already been kicked out of another school for gang affiliation problems. Carlos was given a second chance when he came to my ESL class. I knew something was going on but never knew exactly what it was. I welcomed him as my own child. Soon I discovered that he was a good writer. I always encouraged him to become a writer. I learned a lot about his childhood and how he reunited with his parents after being left in his grandmother's custody in Veracruz, Mexico. Unfortunately, I lost contact with Carlos after he stopped coming to school. I assumed he had dropped out of school. I kept his personal journal as one of my treasures. I reread his personal narratives over and over. I always wondered what happened to him after all of these years. To my surprise, Carlos and I reconnected through social media. He shared with me what happened after he left the school, got taken to jail, and was encouraged to sign self-deportation papers. I also learned how life gave him another chance. Going back to Mexico allowed him to put his life together. He finished his high school and college education. The last time we talked, he shared with me the good news about becoming a father for the first time. I am so glad that Carlos and I are still in touch. When I showed him his personal journal online, he could not believe that I had kept his stories after all of these years. I asked him if he wanted to help me with my writing project and he willingly accepted to be part of it. I also mentioned that I wanted to share his story about racism. Here is what he wrote in 2008:

The day people made my family feel unwelcome

One day my mother, my little sister, and I went to McDonald's. While my little sister was playing around with one of her friends that she met there, at the other side of the fast-food restaurant, there was a white woman eating her meal. My sister kept talking to her friend and joking around with her. The white lady turned around and said to my little sister, "Shut up." My mom got so mad that she became speechless. The only thing that she said was, "vieja grosera." That lady didn't understand what my mom just said to her, but she didn't care. She told my mother that if she didn't like the way things were in this country, then to go back from where she came from. Those words made me, and my family, feel unwelcome, unwanted, and disrespected.

That white lady kept running her mouth. I got so mad that I couldn't take her insults anymore, so I told her, "Shut the fuck up." That lady got so mad that she didn't even get to finish her food. She left shouting, "You are a bunch of spics." We didn't even pay attention to her, so we kept eating like nothing had happened. While she was walking out from the restaurant, some thoughts came to my head. I was thinking if people disrespect you why try to keep all your thoughts in your head when you can make those who disrespect you feel the pain you feel with a couple of words.

Like Carlos, many of my students always shared how some teachers and white students used to remind them to speak English. However, what really struck me the most was to hear Latinx students internalized racism and asked

Spanish-speaking newcomers to stop speaking their heritage language and to start speaking English instead. To counteract those negative comments, I reminded my students to feel proud of their mother tongue since it was part of their cultural identities. I always encouraged them about the importance of navigating in two worlds (Spanish and English) and to be bilingual. Sometimes I also became vulnerable in front of them when sharing my personal testimonios about using Spanish in public and how I responded to people who tried to make me feel bad about my first language. Sharing my personal stories also allowed them to see me not only as a teacher but as a role model. I guess my personal stories and words of empowerment went beyond the ESL classroom.

My classroom was also the place where other Latinx, non-ESL students used to meet. During my second year at this high school, I decided to create an afterschool program that could give Latinx students a sense of belonging. After witnessing how my students felt unwelcome and sometimes profiled as gang members, my ESL students and I decided to start an international club. We used to meet once a month and organized several events in the school and in the community. Again, my classroom became the place where students shared their ideas about community service, Christmas parades, Mother's Day, Hispanic Gala Night, Thanksgiving at nursing homes, Adopt-an-Angel for Christmas, and different fundraisers to support local and international natural disasters. As a community leader, I also founded a non-profit to support Latinx immigrants, many of whom were my students' parents and relatives. This non-profit also allowed my students to become active leaders in their neighborhoods. The international club and the non-profit served as the core to instill in my students a sense of pride for being who they were. I usually reminded them of the importance of their cultural and familial capitals, to work hard for their dreams, and to give back to others. I always promised my students that I wanted to document their experiences. I always wanted other people to know about my students and their stories from their homelands and in the United States.

Although I am no longer teaching ESL students, my role as an educator and social justice advocate has shifted. I now prepare future classroom teachers who are also obtaining an ESL endorsement. My students' stories and my experiences as a former teacher are still vivid in my mind. Not a single day goes by when I do not think about my former students and their relatives. Because of social media, I still keep in touch with many of them. I continue learning about their new families, achievements, travels, birthdays, new jobs, and holidays. I usually visit the town where I used to work and make sure I meet one or two of my former students. I visit their homes and share past memories with them. We are still like a big *familia*. Even though I am no longer teaching them, I still advise them about life, and sometimes parenting. Now I remind them about the importance of supporting their children's education. They continue teaching me about life, hard work, and resiliency. Most of my students came to this country without legal papers and most of them are still living in the shadows as adults and parents. Some others decided to move back to their home countries to pursue higher education and to find decent jobs. My ESL classroom was full of memories from my students. Maybe it is no longer the ESL classroom that it used to be, but what we experienced and shared in that space will never be forgotten.

I wanted to conclude my writing with José, a U.S.-born and raised Mexican-American young adult. He was not an ESL student but a member of the international club. During my last year, he became the president of the club and my mentee. I never realized the impact I caused on José's life until he recently sent me the following message:

High school never really had any meaning until my last years. To me high school was just another school to attend before I went out to the workforce. Not until I started participating in afterschool programs that Mr. Ríos led at the time. Even though Mr. Ríos was not my teacher through my schedule, he was a teacher in my life. With every project or activity, we took on, I learned both about leadership and how to be a generally good person. I can sit and write about every moment we had created at every gathering, but they will all tell the same story, Mr. Ríos was teaching all of us about life. No direct words came out often, but I believe this is why most of his students actually took a lot from him. We didn't notice at the time, but he had all of us under his wings. Being Latino with non-English speaking parents who didn't know much about how school works, which made it kind of tough at some points. That all changed when Mr. Ríos opened his doors to us. I could go and have personal talks and come out brave and ready to take on the world or knock back down to earth and quit messing my life up. Having him at school was critical to my maturing stages. I remember when he taught me a new word in 10th grade. It was humble. He called me humble, and I didn't even know what that meant. After I asked him what it meant, I decided that THAT was how I wanted to live my life. To this day every accomplishment I experience, I think about him in some sort. In high school, accomplishments meant having him around to celebrate or to just work on the next one. We were all special in our own way. We grew up because of him. I don't think there's anyone who left his class without taking something away from him. Mr. Ríos was our father figure at school. The man who we couldn't lie to or hide anything from. Everyone knew about him and knew him well that now it's even weird to call him Doctor Ríos.

Learning from my students through their journals allowed me to see them beyond ELLs, but as vulnerable and brave human beings. I heard amazing and sad stories from them. I learned to become a good listener, a nurse, a lawyer, a confidante, a father figure, a *Tío*, a salsa instructor, a baker, a photographer, and a school and community leader. Being a Latinx teacher, teaching mainly Latinx students, has been my best life journey. My classroom became a healing place.

El aula de inglés como segunda lengua: un lugar de sanación
Montse Feu (Translator)

Llevo los diarios de mis estudiantes conmigo como tesoros personales. A dónde quiera que vaya, intento compartirlos con aquellos estudiantes que serán maestros para que aprendan de las narrativas de mis estudiantes de inglés como segunda lengua.

Me prometí a mis mismo que compartiría las narrativas de mis estudiantes con otras personas. Siempre quise que más individuos aprendieran qué significa ser un inmigrante Latino adolescente en Estados Unidos. En este ensayo comparto las narrativas escritas de tres de mis anteriores estudiantes de inglés como segunda lengua: Sheila, William, and Carlos. Increíblemente, lo que empezó como un proyecto del curso hace diez años, con el que se animaba a los estudiantes a escribir sobre sus historias personales, se convirtieron en artefactos biográficos en una investigación de narrativa,[2] para hacer eco de experiencias personales de los jóvenes latinos escolarizados. Estas narrativas exploran aspectos de los viajes migratorios, la familia, la discriminación y el racismo. Desafortunadamente, dos de mis estudiantes en este ensayo, Sheila and William, fallecieron hace un par de años.

La narrativa de Carlos sobre la discriminación de género y xenofobia me permitió entender mejor el mundo interior de muchos jóvenes latinos y sus familias en este país, especialmente aquellos que no hablan el lenguaje dominante y aquellos que siempre temen ser deportados por no estar documentados legalmente en Estados Unidos. Estos tres estudiantes latinos, como mucho otros, me han dado la fuerza y el poder de escribir este texto.

Cuando llegué a los Estados Unidos como en un intercambio de maestros de mi estimado Panamá hace veinte años, pensaba que iba a enseñar español a hablantes de inglés, como me habían dicho mis amigos antes de venir. Sin embargo, me sorprendió que mis estudiantes eran aprendices de inglés de México, Guatemala, El Salvador, Nicaragua, Honduras, Costa Rica, Panamá, Republica Dominicana, Puerto Rico, Colombia, and Venezuela, así como de Pakistán, India, Vietnam, entre otros muchos países de alrededor del mundo.

Debo confesar que mi llegada al Suroeste norteamericano fue un choque cultural para mí. Aprendí que los conflictos sociales como el racismo y la xenofobia seguían vigentes. Pronto aprendí que las escuelas estaban segregadas racialmente y que las personas de piel oscura y hablantes de español como yo éramos prejuzgados racialmente como "inmigrantes ilegales." Antes de venir a este país, nunca me había cuestionado mi color de pie, o mi acento hispano al hablar inglés, o mi presencia en ciertos lugares. Después de mi llegada, hubo momentos que pensé que mi color de piel y mi acento no me habilitaban como inteligente. A veces me sentí invisible o no bienvenido, especialmente por compañeros o personas de mi ciudad. Muchas veces quise volver a mi país. Me sentía herido y frustrado.

Cuando empecé a enseñar, descubrí que compartía muchas cosas con mis estudiantes además de ser inmigrantes. Nos convertimos en una familia y el salón de español como segunda lengua fue nuestro *hogar*—nuestro espacio de sanación. No hubo ni un día que no aprendiese algo de mis estudiantes y de sus familias. Muchos de mis estudiantes no sabían que me empoderaban no solo como su maestro en la clase, sino también como líder en la comunidad, y un académico latino.

Al principio de impartir clases, me costó que mis estudiantes se involucraran en el aprendizaje del inglés. Me di cuenta de que los estudiantes se sentían angustiados y marginalizados, especialmente cuando otros maestros y estudiantes les decían, "Habla inglés, estás en los Estados Unidos" o "Si quieres hablar español, vuelve a México".

Después de asistir algunas conferencias, aprendí sobre la importancia de incluir un plan de estudios culturalmente relevante en el aula. Inmediatamente me enamoré de autores Latinos tales como Sandra Cisneros, Pat Mora, Isabel Allende, Francisco Jiménez, Gary Soto, y Julia Álvarez. Sus libros me permitieron encontrar lugares comunes con mis estudiantes y desentrañar y analizar de manera crítica nuestras experiencias como inmigrantes. Juntos, descubrimos que no estábamos solos. Al contrario, nuestras lecturas nos llevaron a hablar de nuestras familias y de las expectativas de género, las bandas, el amor, las drogas, los embarazos adolescentes, la pobreza, y las esperanzas. Pudimos aprender como otros inmigrantes y latinos diariamente afrontaban los mismos problemas sociales que nosotros.

El leer sobre racismo, clasismo, inmigración, el aprendizaje del inglés y la educación mediante los ojos de los personajes de estos autores servía para estimular la reflexión de los estudiantes sobre sus experiencias y para explicar sus historias. En el 2008, decidí usar el famoso libro de Sandra Cisneros *A House on Mango Street*, como inspiración para mis estudiantes para que desarrollasen sus propias narrativas. Después de leer y aprender sobre Esperanza y su barrio Latino en Chicago, me di cuenta de lo importante que era para mis estudiantes entender sus historias personales también eran importantes y bienvenidas en mi salón de clase. Cada día, después de leer una o dos viñetas del libro de Cisneros, mis estudiantes escribían sobre sus vidas en sus diarios personales. Escribían sobre sus nombres, sus barrios en los países de origen, así como en Carolina del Norte, un nacimiento en la familia, sus profesores, sus viajes de migración, y las experiencias que les hicieron sentir rechazados en el nuevo país.

Después de las lecturas y de solicitar información de sus diarios personales, decidí que la actividad se convirtiera en un proyecto de escritura. Un día vimos el filme *Freedom Writers* porque quería que tuvieran una idea de que esperaba de sus narrativas. Después de ver la película, Sheila, la estudiante de la que hablaré más tarde dijo, "Ese maestro es como usted, Sr. Ríos." Cuando Sheila lo dijo me di cuenta cuanto me importaban sus narrativas personales, se me hizo un nudo en la garganta y casi lloré.

Cuando terminaron sus narrativas en sus diarios, los llevé a la sala de las computadoras para que pudiesen teclear sus relatos. Fue muy conmovedor ver el entusiasmo de mis estudiantes al convertirse en autores de sus libros, como les había dicho. Mientras tecleaban, fui acercándome por toda la clase y les pedí que incluyeran más detalles en sus relatos.

Cuando terminaron de escribir y editarlos, les enseñé como crear la cubierta delantera y como encuadernarlos. Incluyeron una dedicación y un índice. Otros incluyeron imágenes y pegatinas, así como dibujos y títulos. Cuando terminaron, organicé una fiesta para celebrar los libros. Compramos comida y bebida. Durante la celebración, pedí a los estudiantes que hicieron un círculo y que agarrasen uno de sus relatos para leerlo en voz alta. Cuando leyeron sus textos, todos reímos, reflexionamos, nos hicimos más preguntas y también lloramos. Me acuerdo cuando Verónica, una estudiante mexicana, escribió sobre mí en su dedicatoria. Ella lloró y me hizo llorar al compartir lo agradecida que estaba de que fuera su maestro. Ese año Verónica cumplió quince años. La sorprendimos con un pastel y con refrescos ya que su mamá no pudo costearse una fiesta de quinceañera para ella. Los estudiantes como Verónica y muchos otros han moldeado mi vida como ser humano y como maestro. Guardo los diarios de mis estudiantes desde entonces. Siempre comparto sus relatos personales con otros.

Sheila llegó a los Estados Unidos y empezó en la escuela su primer año en el 2004. Siempre mostraba su alegría y su disposición de aprender un nuevo lenguaje. Era muy inteligente y talentosa. Le encantaba dibujar y decorar. Además, era una bailarina excelente y le encantaba participar en el grupo de baile folclórico mexicano que organicé en la escuela. Después de que se trasladara a México de nuevo con su familia, seguimos en contacto por Facebook por dos años. Sheila compartía fotos de su boda y de sus artesanías. Parecía muy contenta de estar de vuelta en su país natal. Desafortunadamente, el diez de octubre del 2014, otro estudiante me envío un correo con las malas noticias de su fallecimiento después de una operación de corazón. Fue devastador aceptar la partida temprana de Sheila. Siempre estará en mi corazón y en mi pensamiento. Este es el relato de su viaje migratorio en su diario personal cuando era mi estudiante:

Mi viaje a Estados Unidos. [This is Sheila's diary reproduced in the author's contribution not a new text]

Todo pasó tan rápido, después de que mi papá nos dejase para venir a Estados Unidos, mi mamá decidió venir con él. Lo vendió todo, el coche, la ropa, los muebles, todo cuanto teníamos. Finalmente, alquiló la casa, y entonces supimos que había llegado el momento de dejar México y mi vida allí. Como todo pasó muy rápido, no tuvimos tiempo de decir adiós a las personas que amábamos. Un día nos levantamos y mi mamá le dijo a mi hermano, "Nos vamos hoy; nos vamos con vuestro padre. Tenemos que permanecer juntos como la familia que somos".

Ese día subimos al bus que va a Nuevo Laredo. Había una mujer esperándonos. Parecía rara, pero teníamos que ir con ella si queríamos estar con mi papá otra vez. Habló con mi mamá y mi mamá le dijo que todo lo que hacía lo hacía por nosotros, mi hermano y yo, porque nos quería, y porque éramos las personas más importantes en su vida. Al principio, no sabía que estaba pasando hasta que me dijo, "Sheila, tengo que ir de otro modo. Voy a cruzar por el rio al otro lado, pero tú vas con tu hermano, por favor, hija, cuídalo y cuídate". Tuve tanto miedo que no quería dejarla ir, pero no tenía otra elección. Tenía que ser responsable y cuidar de mi hermano.

Ese día, me hice mujer. Mi mamá confiaba en mí y no podía defraudarla. Mi mamá nos abrazó y nos hizo saber lo mucho que nos quería mientras lloraba. Luego se fue. Esos fueron los días más duros para mí y mi hermano, pero me ayudaron a madurar. Ya no era una niña. Era una persona que no solo se protegía a sí misma sino también la vida de mi hermano.

La segunda noche que mi hermano y yo estábamos en Houston, Texas, en casa de mi tío aguardando por las noticias de mi mamá. Lo llamaron para hacerle saber que mi mamá estaba a salvo y que estaba de camino a Houston. Fui tan feliz cuando llegó a casa. Cuando nos vio, empezó a llorar y a besarnos. Nos dijo que nunca más nos dejaría. Era una promesa. Pasamos unos días en Houston, pero luego emprendimos nuestro camino a Carolina del Norte donde nos esperaba nuestro papá.

La historia de inmigración de Sheila era común entre los otros estudiantes de mi clase. Muchos de ellos habían dejado abuelos, familiares, y amigos para reunirse con sus padres, normalmente el padre, quien había dejado el país primero, ahorrado dinero, y había pagado un coyote para que los trajera a Estados Unidos. Se me rompía el corazón al escuchar las historias de mis estudiantes sobre la reunificación con sus padres después de muchos años de separación. Algunos recordaban haberse abrazado y besado a hombres equivocados que habían confundido por sus padres; otros confesaron tener una vida dura con sus padres biológicos puesto que se habían acostumbrado a sus abuelos y los reconocían como sus verdaderos padres.

Una de las experiencias más reveladoras que han impactado mi vida fue escuchar o leer sobre los viajes de inmigración de mis estudiantes y su cruzar peligroso de ríos y fronteras. Leí testimonios de chicas jóvenes que se vistieron como chicos para evitar ser violados por coyotes, de niños vestidos en ropa negra o desnudos para evitar que los oficiales de inmigración los detectaran, de cruzar la frontera con pasaportes falsos, y de ver a personas morir. También leí relatos de pobreza y hambre, de madres solteras, de padres y familiares asesinados, de hermanos mayores que se dejaban atrás, o de funerales de un abuelo u otro familiar al que no podían asistir. Sin embargo, también leí relatos de esperanza y orgullo, especialmente cuando mis estudiantes hablaron sobre sus padres y como apreciaban que se hubieran sacrificado al venir a Estados Unidos. Los estudiantes como William querían ir bien en la escuela como modo de devolver a su madre todos sus esfuerzos para darle una vida mejor.

William era un adolescente mexicano bien parecido. Siempre estaba enamorado. Le gustaba vestir bien. Era muy respetuoso y lleno de energía. Como algunos adolescentes Latinx, también se metió en líos por juntarse con personas equivocadas. Le aconsejaba sobre elecciones de vida, novias y la familia.

Me hice buen amigo de su madre y ella sabía lo mucho que me preocupaba por su hijo. La llamé cuando se metió en problemas en la escuela y ella me llamó cuando William infringió la ley. El viaje de William en este mundo fue muy corto. Solo tenía veintitrés años cuando murió en un accidente de coche el 28 de noviembre de 2015. Me quedé anonadado cuando recibí las noticias en mi celular. Iba a visitar uno de mis antiguos estudiantes y le hice saber la tragedia de William. Cuando fui al velatorio de William, le di el pésame a su madre. Me rompió el corazón ver esta trágica escena. Cuando William murió, ya era padre de un niño de dos años que había tenido con su novia del instituto. Nunca había considerado que uno de los estudiantes más allegados se muriese tan pronto. Me sentí como si estuviera teniendo una pesadilla cuando vie el cuerpo de William en una plataforma de metal con una camisa roja y unos pantalones de mezclilla, con un sombrero mexicano. No puedo borrar esa escena de una madre llorando la muerte de su hijo. William amaba mucho a su madre y a su hermana pequeña. Siempre hablaba con altura de su madre y de su objetivo de estudiar para arquitecto en México. Esto es lo que escribió en su diario personal en el 2008:

Estimado Mr. Ríos,

Me llamó William Hernández. Tengo quince años. Vivo en la ciudad de Asheboro, en Carolina del Norte. Tengo el cabello negro y la piel oscura. Soy una persona honesta que me gusta respetar a los demás y ayudarlos. Me gusta escribir y jugar a fútbol.

Voy a la escuela por la mañana los días de diario. Cuando vuelvo a casa, primero ayudo a mi mamá con las tareas de la casa y luego como. Vivo con mi mamá y mi hermana. Nos ayudamos. Cuando acabo de ayudar a mi mamá, a veces hago mi tarea de la escuela y escucho música. Como mi papá no vive con nosotros, vivimos en un apartamento pequeño.

Ahora mi mamá tiene un novio, que quiere casarse con ella y llevarnos a Charlotte, para tener una mejor vida. Mi madre es muy trabajadora y honesta. Me ayuda mucho. La quiero mucho. Mi hermana tiene seis años. Ella va a la guardería. La quiero mucho porque es genial. Bueno a veces es tremenda porque agarro mi lugar y ahora todas las personas dicen que es tan adorable y todo eso, así que ya no soy yo el adorable. De todos modos, estoy orgullos de tener esta familia. Esto es todo sobre mí y mi bonita familia.

Estimado Mr. Ríos,

Mi mamá se llama Belén y tiene treinta y seis años. Ella es una madre trabajadora. Le gusta cuidar de las personas mayores, así las personas la podrán ayudar. Lo que más me gusta de mi mamá era que se enfada por todo. Es una persona honesta.

Trabaja en una fábrica, pero su salario es poco. Por ello, tiene que trabajar mucho para sus hijos. Nos quiere mucho, y todo lo que quiere es una vida mejor para nosotros. Le gusta vestir bien pero no para presumir. Lo hace porque así es ella, y ella es muy hermosa.

La única cosa que mi mamá quiere es ser feliz. Quiere casarse con su novio Alberto porque él es una buena persona. Quiere a mi mamá y nos cuida, pero especialmente a mi hermana. Mi madre quiere lo mejor y pienso que estará orgullosa si termino el instituto y me gradúo.

Mi mamá vino hace seis o siete años. Desde entonces, ha trabajado para ahorrar dinero y enviarlo a México donde construir una casa y tener un lugar para una vida mejor.

William se graduó del instituto y siguió trabajando en una fábrica de muebles con otros compañeros Latinx. Desafortunadamente, se separó de la madre de su hijo y empezó a salir con otra chica. Como William, muchos jóvenes Latinx pronto se dieron cuenta que sus deseos de asistir a la universidad eran irrealizables pero su estado migratorio. Como resultado, muchos Latinx no documentados acababan trabajando en fábricas, en restaurantes de comida rápida, en la construcción, y en jardinería. Otros decidieron no terminar el bachillerato por falta de un sistema que los apoye y que les ayude a lidiar las bajas expectativas de la sociedad y de la escuela. Siempre me preocupaba cuando se me decía que un estudiante había decidido no seguir en la escuela. A veces mis estudiantes me mentían sobre sus decisiones de dejar la escuela porque sabían lo mucho que me disgustaba la idea. Les inculcaba que debían seguir en la escuela y obtener su bachillerato. Me usaba como ejemplo para que estuvieran enfocados en sus objetivos. Compartí mi voluntad de inscribirme en una maestría en este país y cuantos años esperé a que se me considerase para pagar la matrícula de residente. Algunos escucharon mis consejos, mientras otros, como Carlos, les costaba aguantar los obstáculos sociales y de la vida en general.

Carlos era el hijo que me hubiera gustado tener. Me recordaba mucho a mi hermano mayor. Cuando vino al instituto, ya lo habían corrido de otra escuela por su asociación con una banda. A Carlos le dieron una segunda oportunidad cuando vino a mi clase de inglés como segunda lengua. Sabía que algo pasaba, pero no sabía exactamente que era. Lo recibí como a un hijo propio. Pronto descubrí que era un buen escritor. Siempre le alenté a que fuera escritor. Aprendí mucho sobre su infancia y como se reunió con sus padres después de que lo hubieran dejado con su abuela en Veracruz, México. Desafortunadamente, perdí el contacto con Carlos después de que dejara de venir a la escuela. Asumí que había dejado los estudios. Guardé su diario personal como uno de mis tesoros. Leí sus narrativas personales una y otra vez. Siempre me pregunté que había sido de él después de tantos años. Sorprendentemente, reconecté con Carlos mediante las redes sociales. Me explicó que había pasado después de dejar los estudios, lo llevaron a la cárcel y se le incitó a que firmara los documentos para una deportación voluntaria. También aprendí que la vida le dio otra oportunidad. El volver a México le permitió recomponer su vida. Terminó el bachillerato y una licenciatura. La última vez que hablamos, me dio las buenas noticias de que había sido padre por primera vez. Estoy muy contento de que sigamos en contacto. Cuando le mostré su diario personal, no podía creer que había guardado sus historias todos estos años. Le pregunté si quería ayudarme con mi proyecto de escritura y acepto de buen grado. También le dije que quería compartir su historia sobre el racismo. Esto es lo que escribió en el 2008:

El día que a mi familia la hicieron sentir incómoda

Un día fui con mi madre y mi hermana pequeña al McDonald's. Mientras que mi hermanita jugaba con unos amigos que se encontró allí, había una señora blanca comiendo su comida al otro lado del restaurante de comida rápida. Mi hermana seguía hablando con su amiga y haciendo bromas con ella. La señora se giró y le dijo a mi hermana, "Cállese". Mi mamá se enfadó tanto que se quedó sin habla. La única cosa que le dijo fue, "Vieja grosera". La señora no entendió lo que le había dicho mi mamá, pero ni siquiera le importó. Le dijo que, si no le gustaban las cosas en este país, se podía ir de donde fuera. Esas palabras nos hicieron sentir mal recibidos, indeseables, y vilipendiados.

La señora seguía criticando. Me enfadé tanto que ya no pude aguantar sus insultos, así que le dije, "Cállese de una puta vez". Esa señora se enfadó tanto que ni tan solo terminó su comida. Se marchó gritando, "Son una pandilla de sudacas". Ni le prestamos atención y seguimos comiendo como si nada hubiera pasado. Mientras se iba del restaurante, me vinieron unos pensamientos a la mente. Pensé que, si alguien te falta al respecto, para qué guardarte tus pensamientos cuando puedes hacerles sufrir la pena que sientes con un par de palabras.

Así como Carlos, muchos de mis estudiantes compartieron como algunos maestros y estudiantes blancos les recordaban que tenían que hablar en inglés. Sin embargo, lo que me afectó más fuer escuchar el racismo internalizado de los estudiantes Latinx cuando pedían a los recién llegados que dejaran de hablar su lenguaje de herencia y que hablaran inglés. Para contrarrestar esos comentarios negativos, les recordaba a mis estudiantes que se sintieran orgullosos de su lengua nativa puesto que era parte de su identidad cultural.

Siempre les alenté sobre la importancia de hacerse camino en dos mundos (español e inglés) y de ser bilingüe. A veces me mostré vulnerable y les conté de experiencias personales de haber hablado español en público y como había respondido a las personas que me habían hecho sentir mal sobre mi primera lengua. El hecho de compartir mis experiencias personales les permitió verme no solo como su maestro, pero también como un modelo. Supongo que mis historias personales y mis palabras de aliento fueron más allá de las clases de inglés como segunda lengua.

Mi clase también era un lugar de encuentro para otros estudiantes Latinx, aunque no fueran estudiantes de inglés como segunda lengua. Durante mi segundo año en este instituto, decidí crear un programa extracurricular que diera a los estudiantes Latinx un sentimiento de pertenencia. Puesto que había visto que algunos de mis estudiantes se sentían mal recibidos cuando se les veía como miembros de bandas, decidimos con mis estudiantes empezar un club internacional. Nos reuníamos una vez al mes y organizábamos varios eventos en la escuela y en la comunidad. Una vez más, mi salón se convirtió en el lugar donde mis estudiantes compartían sus ideas sobre el voluntariado a la comunidad, desfiles de Navidad, el día de la madre, la gala Hispana, el Día de Acción de Gracias en residencias de ancianos, el programa Adopta un Ángel en Navidad, y otras formas de recolectar fondos para apoyar desastres naturales locales e internacionales. Como líder de la comunidad, también fundé una organización sin animo de lucro para apoyar a los inmigrantes Latinx, mucho de los cuales fueron los padres y los familiares de mis estudiantes. Esta organización también permitió a mis estudiantes convertirse en líderes activos de sus barrios. El club internacional y la organización fueron los pilares para fomentar en mis estudiantes un sentimiento de orgullo de ser quien eran. Usualmente les recordaba la importancia de su capital cultural y familiar, que lucharan por sus sueños, y que dieran oportunidades a otros. Siempre les prometí a mis estudiantes que quería documentar sus experiencias. Siempre quise que otras personas supieran sobre mis estudiantes y sus historias de sus países de origen y en los Estados Unidos.

Aunque ya no enseño a estudiantes de inglés como segunda lengua, mi papel como educador y defensor de la justicia social ha cambiado. Ahora preparo a futuros maestros que también preparan su para obtener sus credenciales. Las historias y las experiencias de mis estudiantes siguen vivas en mi recuerdo. No hay un día que pase que no piense en mis antiguos estudiantes y sus familiares. Gracias a las redes sociales, sigo en contacto con muchos de ellos. Sigo aprendiendo sobre sus familias, logros, viajes, cumpleaños, trabajos nuevos, y vacaciones.

Normalmente visito la ciudad donde trabajé y me aseguro de encontrarme con alguno de mis antiguos estudiantes. Visito sus casas y compartimos memorias. Aun somos una gran familia. Aunque ya no les imparto clase, aún les doy consejo sobre su vida, y sobre la crianza de sus hijos. Ahora les recuerdo la importancia de respaldar la educación de sus hijos. Me siguen enseñando sobre su vida, su trabajo duro y su resiliencia. Muchos de mis estudiantes vinieron a este país indocumentados y como adultos y padres siguen viviendo en la sombra.

Otros prefirieron volver a sus países de origen, estudiar una carrera y encontrar trabajos dignos. Mi clase de inglés como segunda lengua, estaba llena de memorias de mis estudiantes. Quizás ya no es la clase que solía ser, pero lo que experimentamos y compartimos en ese lugar no se nos olvidará.

Querría concluir mi escrito con José, un joven nacido en Estados Unidos y criado como un mexicanoamericano. No era estudiante de inglés como segunda lengua, sino miembro del club internacional. Durante mi último año, fue el presidente del club y mi tutelado. Nunca supe del efecto que causé en la vida de José hasta que recientemente me envió este mensaje:

La escuela secundaria nunca tuvo ningún sentido hasta mis últimos años. Para mi el instituto no era más que otra escuela a que debía asistir para poder empezar a trabajar. Fue así hasta que empecé los programas extracurriculares que el señor Ríos lideraba en ese momento. Aunque el Sr. Ríos no fue mi maestro de ninguna de mis clases, fue un maestro de mi vida. Con cada proyecto o actividad que nos hacíamos cargo, aprendí sobre liderazgo y como ser una buena persona. Me puedo sentar y escribir sobre cada momento que creamos en nuestras reuniones, pero todos dirán lo mismo, el Sr. Ríos nos enseñaba a todos sobre la vida. No fueron palabras explicitas, pero creo que eso precisamente era lo que muchos de sus estudiantes se llevaron con ellos. No nos dimos cuenta entonces, pero nos tenía a todos bajo su ala. Por ser Latino y por tener padres que no hablaban inglés, no sabíamos como funcionaba la escuela y eso podía ser difícil a veces. Todo eso cambió cuando el Sr. Ríos nos abrió sus puertas. Podía ir y hablarle de mis asuntos personales y salir valiente y preparado para enfrentarme al mundo, tocar de pies a tierra y dejar de complicarme la vida. Tenerlo en la secundaria fue fundamental en mi proceso de maduración. Me acuerdo cuando me enseño una palabra nueva en el décimo grado. Era la palabra modesto. Me llamó modesto y no sabía qué significaba. Después de preguntarle qué significaba, decidí que eso era como quería vivir mi vida. Hasta hoy, cada logro que experimento, pienso en él de algún modo. En la secundaria, los logros eran compartidos con él y los celebrábamos o simplemente nos poníamos a trabajar en el próximo objetivo. Todos eran especiales para nosotros. Crecimos gracias a él. No creo que

hubiera nadie que dejase su clase sin haber aprendido algo. Era nuestra figura pater-
nal en la escuela. Era el hombre al que no podíamos mentir o esconder nada. Todos
lo conocíamos y lo conocíamos bien que llamarlo ahora doctor suena raro.

El aprender de mis estudiantes con sus diarios me permitió verlos más allá
de estudiantes de inglés como segunda lengua, como seres humanos vulne-
rables y valientes. Escuché sus historias increíbles y tristes. Aprendí a ser un
buen oyente, un enfermero, un abogado, un confidente, una figura paterna,
un tío, un instructor de salsa, un panadero, un fotógrafo, y un líder escolar y
comunitario. Haber sido un maestro Latinx y haber enseñado a estudiantes
Latinx ha sido el mejor viaje vital. Mi clase se convirtió en un lugar de sanación.

Notes

1. Creswell, J. W. and Poth, C. N. *Qualitative inquiry & research design: Choosing among five approaches* (4th ed.). Thousand Oaks, California: Sage Publications, Inc., 2018.
2. Creswell, J. W. and Poth, C. N. *Qualitative inquiry & research design: Choosing among five approaches* (4th ed.). Thousand Oaks, California: Sage Publications, Inc., 2018.

· 1 3 ·

AMELIA COTTER

"The Love of Strangers," by Amelia Cotter portrays the relationship between a young Mexican boy and a detention center worker in Texas in 2016. The story is written by author Amelia Cotter because the worker at the detention center did not want to be identified.

The Love of Strangers[1]

Unaccompanied Children are placed under the Office for Refugee Resettlement (ORR)/Division of Children Services (DCS) after being apprehended by the Department of Homeland Security (DHS) for having no lawful immigration status in the United States, not having attained 18 years of age, and having no parent or legal guardian in the United States available to provide care and physical custody (Michelson 2017: 108).[2]

Lupe sees Luis arrive alone and afraid, no older than seven or eight. His future is uncertain, and his potential abounds. Lupe knows Luis has no idea what is going to happen next and that he does not understand if he's in trouble. He is surrounded by strangers—are they good people, there to help? There to punish, convict? Lupe is sure he's heard stories. She smiles at him knowing he must have so many questions. Do they care about him, and the other children there like him? Or are there so many children to care for that there is no love left over for one little boy like himself?

Lupe tells him that he will be staying here, at the detention center, until he can be sent back home or with a sponsor. She focuses on smiling at him and explaining that he will be staying here until a relative is able to take custody of him, but it may take them and their volunteer lawyers a long time to find a family member willing or able to claim him. She asks him if he feels alone and afraid. Luis nods his head, "Yes." She tells him that members of his family may also feel alone and afraid, and he must wait but it doesn't mean he has been forgotten.

Lupe has taken charge of his care. He must be courageous and patient, she tells him. It could be days, weeks, months, years that he might wait for word from a relative. She says that he has already been on a long and difficult journey, and he is a very brave boy. If he could make it through that journey, then he can make it through this one as well.

Many here speak Spanish, but Lupe tells him that he may not, unless in simple sentences or phrases that everyone here can understand. Luis will be taught English and math and other subjects he would normally learn in school. Luis may not touch anyone, and not allow himself to be touched by anyone else.

Lupe imagines that all Luis really wants is a hug. He chooses not to speak at all.

Luis is quiet. He seems to be calculating the goodness in the people around him, in preparation for his impending fate.

But Lupe is always nice to him. He doesn't seem to understand everything she says at first, but he seems to like her. Lupe hopes he feels protected when she is around. She wants him to feel like he matters. They cannot touch but Lupe tries to warm his heart with her smile and her encouraging words.

She makes sure he eats every day. She helps him learn his subjects, like he would at school, and helps him stay in good spirits, like he would if he lived in a real home.

They color together. Lupe brings him pictures of animals: armadillos, ants, bears, butterflies. Lupe picks out a crayon. "My favorite color is blue," she says.

"Mine, too," Luis replies in his newly burgeoning voice. Her eyes light up when he speaks. There are many blue crayons, and many pictures at the center to color, and so their time there passes.

In fact, 2 years pass. Lupe updates Luis regularly on the progress of the center's volunteer lawyers in finding a family member. One day, she has news: he is finally going home.

Luis seems afraid when she shares the news with him. An uncle, one he barely seems to remember, will be taking custody of him. The center is not home. No, he is going home.

Lupe says that he should not feel alone or afraid. She will go with him to meet his uncle. She'll be on the plane with him and will be there with him every step of the way.

On the plane, Luis cries uncontrollably. He seems embarrassed and sad and says that he feels both alone and afraid. Lupe does all she can to comfort him. She has spent 2 years trying to be strong for him and trying to help him be strong. She reassures him that none of this is his fault. Lupe tells him again that he has been a very brave boy. She will miss him so much.

They meet his uncle at the airport. His tries to embrace his nephew, but Luis stands behind Lupe as if to feel safer. This is the first time that Luis would have experienced a real hug in such a long time, but Lupe thinks that his uncle must look like a stranger to him.

There is paperwork to be done. Lupe has his uncle sign a stack of forms. Seizing his chance, Luis puts his arms around Lupe as tightly as he can. Lupe turns around, takes Luis by the arms, bends down, and hugs him back. She tells him that he must go with this man, his uncle, and be reunited with his family. She was once a stranger to him, too, but now they're friends. And his uncle may seem like a stranger to him now, but that soon may also change.

His uncle takes him by the hand. In his other hand, Luis clutches his small suitcase. As Lupe watches Luis depart once again into the unknown, she wonders if she will ever see him again.

Luis never takes his eyes off of her as he walks away, not until he is completely out of sight.

El amor de extraños³
Blanca P. Tovar Frias (Translator)

Los niños no acompañados son tutelados por la Oficina de Reasentamiento para Refugiados "Refugee Resettlement (ORR)" de la División de Servicios para Niños "Division of Children Services (DCS)", después de ser arrestados por el Departamento de Seguridad Nacional "Department of Homeland Security (DHS)" por no tener un estado migratorio legal en los Estados Unidos, no haber alcanzado los 18 años de edad, y no tener padres o tutor legal asequible para proveer atención y protección física (Michelson 2017: 108).

Lupe lo ve llegar solo y asustado a Luis, no tiene más de siete u ocho años. Su futuro es incierto y su potencial es abundante. Lupe sabe que Luis no tiene idea de qué le pasará y no sabe si se ha metido en un lío. Está rodeado de extraños - ¿Son buenas personas, para ayudarlo? ¿Para castigarlo, o condenarlo? Lupe está segura de que ha escuchado historias. Ella le sonríe sabiendo que debe tener muchas preguntas. ¿Se preocupan por él y por los otros niños como él? ¿O hay tantos niños que cuidar que no queda amor para un niño como él?

Lupe le dice que se quedará aquí, en el centro de detención hasta que lo pueden mandar a su casa o a casa de un patrocinador. Lupe se concentra en sonreírle y explicarle que permanecerá aquí hasta que algún familiar sea capaz de tutelarlo. Pero esto les va a tomar tiempo a ellos y a sus abogados voluntarios puesto que se debe encontrar un miembro de la familia dispuesto o capaz de reclamarlo. Ella le pregunta si se siente sólo o asustado. Luis asiente con la cabeza. Ella le dice que los miembros de su familia quizá se sientan solos y asustados también, y debe esperarlos, pero esto no quiere decir que lo han olvidado.

Lupe se ha hecho cargo de su cuidado. Le dice que debe ser valiente y paciente. Podrían ser días, semanas, meses, o años hasta que él escuche noticias de un pariente. Le dice que ha hecho ya un largo y difícil viaje y él es un muchacho muy valiente. Si él pudo superar ese viaje, entonces él puede superar esto también.

Muchos aquí hablan español, pero Lupe le dicen que no debe, a menos que sean oraciones y frases simples que todos aquí puedan entender. Luis aprenderá inglés, matemáticas y otros temas que él normalmente aprendería en la escuela. No debe tocar a nadie y no debe permitir que nadie lo toque a él.

Lupe piensa que todo lo que quiere Luis es un abrazo. Luis decide no hablar en absoluto.

Lupe siempre es amable con él. No parece entender todo lo que ella le dice al principio, pero parece que le gusta. Lupe espera que se sienta protegido cuando ella está cerca. Lo hace sentir querido. No se pueden tocar. Lupe intenta confortarlo con su sonrisa y sus alentadoras palabras.

Se asegura de que coma cada día. Lo ayuda a aprender sus temas, como lo haría en la escuela y lo ayuda a mantener un buen ánimo como el que tendría si viviera un hogar verdadero.

Colorean juntos. Lupe le trae fotos de animales: armadillos, hormigas, osos, mariposas. Lupe escoge un crayón. "Mi color favorito es azul", dice Ella.

"El mío también", contesta Luis con una recién y floreciente voz. Los ojos de Lupe se iluminan cuando él habla. Hay muchos crayones azules y muchas imágenes en el centro para colorear, y así pasa su tiempo ahí.

De hecho, pasan dos años. Lupe le informa regularmente sobre el progreso de los abogados voluntarios del centro para encontrar a un miembro de la familia. Un día, Lupe tiene noticias: finalmente Luis se va a casa.

Luis parece asustado al escuchar a Lupe. Un tío, uno que apenas recuerda, se hará cargo de su tutela. El centro no es un hogar. No, él se va a casa.

Lupe le dice que no se sienta solo o asustado. Irá con él a encontrar a su tío. Estará en el avión con él, y estará ahí con él a cada paso del camino.

En el avión, Luis llora incontrolablemente. Parece avergonzado y triste y dice que se siente solo y temeroso. Ella hace todo lo que puede para consolarlo. Por dos años, Lupe ha sido fuerte por él y ha tratado de ayudarlo a ser fuerte. Le asegura que nada de lo que ha pasado ha sido su culpa. Dice que él ha sido un niño muy valiente. Lo extrañará mucho.

Conocen a su tío en el aeropuerto. Su tío intenta abrazar a su sobrino, pero Luis se esconde detrás de ella como para sentirse protegido. Es el primer abrazo verdadero que Luis hubiera recibido en mucho tiempo, pero Lupe puede entender que su tío le parezca un extraño.

Hay papeleo por hacer. Ella indica a su tío el montón de formularios que hay que firmar. Aprovechando la oportunidad, Luis la abraza tan fuerte como puede. Lupe se voltea, lo toma por los brazos, se inclina, y lo abraza también. Debe irse con el señor, su tío, y reunirse con la familia. Una vez, ella también fue una extraña para él y ahora son amigos. Su tío puede parecerle un extraño ahora, pero eso también puede cambiar pronto.

Su tío lo toma de la mano. Con su otra mano, él agarra su pequeña maleta. Antes de partir una vez más hacia lo desconocido, Lupe se pregunta si lo volverá a ver.

Luis nunca aparta la vista de Lupe al alejarse, no hasta que está completamente fuera de su vista.

Notes

1. Montse Feu would like to dedicate this story to Lupe and to those who work at detention centers and try to heal with their loving care.
2. Michelson, Seth. *Dreaming America*. Silver Spring: Settlement House, 2017.
3. Montse Feu quisiera dedicar este relato a Lupe y aquellas personas que trabajan en centros de detención y que intentan sanar con su cariño.

ABOUT THE AUTHORS

Co-Editors

Montse Feu is an associate professor of Hispanic Studies at Sam Houston State University. She migrated to the USA in 2005 and is a first-generation scholar. She recovers the literary history of the Spanish Civil War exile in the United States, U.S., Hispanic periodicals, and migration literature at large. She has published 10 chapters and 10 articles in peer-reviewed publications. Feu is the author of *Correspondencia personal y política de un anarcosindicalista exiliado: Jesús González Malo (1943–1965)* (Universidad de Cantabria, 2016) and *Fighting Fascist Spain*, (University of Illinois Press, 2020). She is co-editor of *Writing Revolution: Hispanic Anarchism in the United States* (University of Illinois Press, 2019). She is the director of the Recovery Digital project *Fighting Fascist Spain – The Exhibits*. Feu is board member for the Recovering the U. S. Hispanic Literary Heritage and treasurer for the Research Society for American Periodicals.
Email: mmf017@shsu.edu
Postal Address: 7 Moonseed Place, The Woodlands Texas, 77381, USA.

Amanda Venta, Ph.D. is an Associate Professor in the Department of Psychology at the University of Houston. Her research focuses on attachment between parents and children and how the quality of these attachments relates to mental health and well-being at biological and behavioral levels. Her interest in attachment disruptions spurred her focus on Central American immigration, a context in which families are often separated for long periods of time. She is a first generation American herself and has provided psychological services to unaccompanied immigrant minors in the custody of the Office of Refugee Resettlement since 2012, including graduate students in that experience since 2015. Her research has been funded by the National Institute of Mental Health, the National Institute of Minority Health and Health Disparities, and the American Psychological Foundation. She has authored or co-authored three books, 16 chapters, and more than 80 manuscripts. Notable among these contributions are an edited volume textbook entitled *Developmental Psychopathology* for students of psychology and articles published in the *Journal of the American Academy of Child and Adolescent Psychiatry*, the *Journal of Clinical Child and Adolescent Psychology*, *Psychological Assessment*, and *Attachment and Human Development*.

Email: aventa@uh.edu

Postal Address: The University of Houston, Health 1, 4849 Calhoun Road, Room 373, Houston, TX 77204-6022

Contributors

Maria Baños Jordan is a native Houstonian, and graduate of the University of Houston with a degree in Sociology. She is the President and Founder of the Texas Familias Council. The Council has served the Houston region since 2011 by advocating for and guiding local Latino, immigrant, and underserved communities. She is the daughter of a Cuban refugee and Mexican immigrant and has professionally served vulnerable families in the Houston region through social service institutions since 1995. Maria initiated the first Latino-focused community development effort in Montgomery County, TX, and has created numerous projects guiding women's and Latino progress. Maria created The Conroe Historias Project, an intercultural biography compilation authored by local Latino youth, and archived in the Montgomery County Memorial Library System in 2011. She leads disaster and crisis response efforts for underserved areas. In 2013 Maria received a Texas State Senate Proclamation for her efforts and was appointed to the Montgomery County Historical Commission. She leads the Texas HOPE Consortium to engage the region's social service professionals on issues of diversity and inclusion. She has served on local medical, historical, and legal nonprofit boards of directors, and has authored numerous articles on community issues.

Email: texasfamilias@outlook.com

Postal Address: 6518 Upper Lake Dr.   Kingwood, TX 77346

Contribution: "Spanish Silencio/"

Cassandra Bailey is a sixth-year doctoral candidate in the clinical psychology program with a forensic emphasis at Sam Houston State University. Her current research interests are broadly in the areas of immigration, forensics, and diversity issues. For her master's thesis, she examined how immigration court impacts the mental health of Spanish-speaking youth, a topic expanded upon in her dissertation in which she examined how legal, religious, and social support may function as points of intervention to mitigate distress associated with court. For her major area paper, she explored the extant literature regarding how bilingualism affects tests of cognitive abilities. Cassandra is passionate about clinical work with immigrant populations, with a specific focus on Latinx Spanish-speakers.

Email: cab115@shsu.edu

Postal Address: 61 Acacia Street, Clearwater Beach, FL 33767

Contribution: "Growing Up Too Fast."

Melissa Briones immigrated at the age of three to the United States with her family from Gomez Palacio, Durango, Mexico. She grew up in the Rio Grande Valley, a region in the United States that is separated from Mexico by the Rio Grande river. For much of her childhood she lived in this country as an undocumented immigrant which has fueled her commitment to underserved and underrepresented populations. She completed a Bachelor of Arts in Psychology locally at the University of Texas-Rio Grande Valley and a Master of Arts degree in Clinical Psychology at Sam Houston State University. She is currently a doctoral student in the Counseling Psychology program at the University of North Texas.

Email: melissabriones@my.unt.edu

Postal Address: 3005 Augusta Rd., Apt C., Denton, TX 76207

Contribution: With Alfonso Mercado, Abigail Nunez-Saenz, Paola Quijano, and Andy Torres, "Buscando un destino."

Yessica Colin obtained a Psychology bachelor's degree from Sam Houston State University where she graduated *cum laude* in 2019. Her research interests are broadly in the areas of assessment and intelligence. She seeks to create decision support applications that will help clinical experts with mental health diagnoses and screenings. During her undergraduate career, Yessica was involved in the *Youth and Family Studies Lab*, a lab that studies psychopathology among recently immigrated adolescents, where she had the opportunity to become involved in research. She has presented her research at the *SHSU Undergraduate Research Symposium*, which was subsequently presented at the *Texas Psychological Association's* annual conference and won a student paper award. As an undergraduate, Yessica has also written a manuscript (Yessica the first author) under the guidance of her lab's principal investigator— Dr. Amanda Venta. She is currently working at a behavioral healthcare facility and in the future, she wishes to enroll in a cognitive science program.

Email: colinyessica@gmail.com

Postal Address: 934 Crestmont Place Loop Missouri City, TX 77489

Contribution: "Camila."

Amelia Cotter is an author, storyteller, and award-winning poet with a special interest in history and folklore. She is the author of several books for adults and children, and her poetry and short fiction have appeared in journals like *Barren Magazine*, *Frogpond*, *Modern Haiku*, *The Heron's Nest*, *tinywords*, and many others. Her work often explores the themes of alienation, isolation, and anxiety. Amelia lives and writes in Chicago but is originally from Maryland, where she earned a degree in German and History from Hood College. She has appeared on various radio and television programs, and regularly presents at conferences and events. Amelia is a member of the Society of Midland Authors. Amelia's official website is www.ameliacotter.com.

Email: ameliamcotter@gmail.com

Postal Address: 3130 N. Lake Shore Dr., Apt. 1806 Chicago, IL 60657

Contribution: "The Love of Strangers."

Montse Feu is an associate professor of Hispanic Studies at Sam Houston State University. She recovers the literary history of the Spanish Civil War exile in the United States, U.S., Hispanic periodicals, and migration literature at large. She migrated to the USA in 2005 and is a first-generation scholar. She is the author of *Correspondencia personal y política de un anarco-sindicalista exiliado: Jesús González Malo (1943–1965)* (Universidad de Cantabria, 2016) and *Fighting Fascist Spain*, (University of Illinois Press, 2020), She is co-editor of *Writing Revolution: Hispanic Anarchism in the United States*

(University of Illinois Press, 2019). She is board member for the Recovering the U. S. Hispanic Literary Heritage and for the Research Society for American Periodicals.

Email: mmf017@shsu.edu

Postal Address: 7 Moonseed Place, The Woodlands Texas, 77381, USA.

Contribution: With Amanda Venta, "Introduction: Serving Refugee Children and their Families."

Ana M. Fores Tamayo is ABD in Comparative Literature from New York University. Being an academic not paid enough for her trouble, she wanted instead to do something that mattered: work with asylum seekers. She advocates for marginalized refugee families from Mexico and Central America. This work is heart wrenching yet satisfying. It is also quite humbling. Her labor has eased her own sense of displacement, being a child refugee, always trying to find home. She has been at the forefront of the *Refugee Support Network* in Dallas, participating in its *pro se* asylum workshops since their inception in 2014. She also volunteers remotely with *Lawyers for Good Government* in Matamoros. She was a panelist at the University of North Texas' Refugee Summit & Santa Fe's Conference for Applied Anthropology, *"Witnessing" the Migration Crisis Across Borders*. In parallel, poetry is Fores Tamayo's escape: she has published in *The Raving Press, Indolent Books, Laurel Review* and many other anthologies and journals, here and internationally, online and in-print. Her poetry in translation & photography have been exhibited in art fairs and galleries too. Writing is a catharsis from the cruelty yet ecstasy of her work. Through it, she keeps tilting at windmills.

Email: mayari@mac.com

Postal Address: 1714 Falcon Drive Keller, TX 76248

Contribution: "Elegy to a Refugee Girl," "Oda a una niña refugiada."

Dr. Luz M. Garcini, Ph.D., MPH, is an Assistant Professor at the Center for Research to Advance Community Health (ReACH) at the University of Texas Health Science Center San Antonio, and a Faculty Scholar at the Baker Institute for Public Policy at Rice University. Dr. Garcini obtained her doctoral degree in Clinical Psychology from San Diego State University/University of California San Diego (SDSU/UCSD) and a combined Master of Public Health (MPH) Epidemiology from the SDSU Graduate School of

Public Health. Broadly, Dr. Garcini's research focuses on identifying, understanding, and addressing the health needs of Latinx immigrant families.

Her line of research (*Project Voices*) is a combination of community efforts and research studies which for the past 12 years have generated scientific evidence to document and address the complex health needs of undocumented Latinxs. Her commitment to research aimed at informing social justice is evident in her track record of publications, presentations, awards received, and funding allocated. Her work has received widespread national and international media coverage in avenues such as Univision, Telemundo, CBS, U.S. News and World Report, and Global News Report.

Email: garcini@uthscsa.edu

Postal Address: Center for Research to Advance Community Health (ReACH). UT Health. San Antonio. Joe R. and Teresa Lozano Long School of Medicine. 7703 Floyd Curl Drive, San Antonio, Texas.

Contribution: With Martin La Roche, "An Undocumented Journey in Search of a Heart."

Estrella Godinez is a graduate student at Sam Houston State University. Ms. Godinez is pursuing a master's degree in clinical Mental Health Counseling. She has published in *The Measure: An Undergraduate Research Journal* studying the connection between parental attachment and risky sexual behavior in adolescents. She has presented her undergraduate research in the form of a poster presentation at the Texas Psychological Association Annual Convention in 2017. Ms. Godinez has contributed to research publications pertaining to the mental health of immigrated youth in schools. She has conducted research on the developmental psychopathology of adolescents with borderline personality disorder.

Email: Edg015@shsu.edu, stargodinez@icloud.com

Postal Address: 7005 Allen Dr., Conroe, TX 77304

Contribution: "A Yearning Desire," "Un deseo anhelante."

Martin La Roche, Ph.D., has been Director of Psychology Training at the Boston Children's' Hospital at Martha Eliot (which is the oldest standing community health center in the United States) for the last twenty-five years, where he treats an inner city and culturally diverse community, many who are undocumented immigrants. In addition, he trains and supervises doctoral level psychologists, social workers and psychiatrists. In addition, Dr. La Roche is an Associate Professor in Psychology at the Harvard Medical School/Boston Children's Hospital and has over 100 publications/presentations and two books "Cultural Psychotherapy: Theory, Methods and Practice" and "Towards a Global and Cultural Psychotherapy." He is regularly invited to present in national and international conferences. He has received many research/academic awards from community, academic and state institutions. He also co-chaired the Committee of Ethnic Minority Affairs at Massachusetts for many years.

Email: Martin.Laroche@childrens.harvard.edu

Postal Address: Martin La Roche, Ph.D. 49 Hancock St. Suite 104. Cambridge MA. 02139.

Contribution: With Luz M. Garcini, "An Undocumented Journey in Search of a Heart."

Dr. Alfonso Mercado, originally from Los Angeles, California, currently is an Associate Professor in the Department of Psychological Science and Department of Psychiatry in the School of Medicine at the University of Texas-Rio Grande Valley. He is a Licensed Psychologist and a National Register Health Service Psychologist. Dr. Mercado's current research lab focuses on Latino mental health, trauma and immigration, personality, substance abuse, and multicultural interventions. He is President-Elect Designate for the Texas Psychological Association and was recently elected to the Committee on Rural Health at the American Psychological Association. He teaches and collaborates routinely with the Universidad de Guadalajara in Mexico and Universidad Central de Ecuador in Quito. Dr. Mercado was the recipient of Faculty Excellence in Sustainability Education Award at the UTRGV and was awarded the Knowledge Award for Excellence in Education and Research by the American Association of Intellectual and Developmental Disabilities-Texas Chapter. He was also recognized by the Texas Psychological Association for Outstanding Contribution to Education Award and the Psychologist of the Year award in 2019 for his efforts in immigration and mental health at the U.S.-Mexico Border.

Email: alfonso.mercado@utrgv.edu

Postal Address: 1201 W. University Drive, Edinburg, Texas 78539

Contribution: With Briones and al, "Buscando un destino."

Seth Michelson is Associate Professor of Spanish at Washington and Lee University, where he founded and now directs the Center for Poetic Research. His scholarship focuses on poetry and state violence in the hemispheric Americas, and he has published peer-reviewed book chapters, articles, essays, and reviews on carcerality, poetry, and aesthetics in leading venues in the US, Argentina, Italy, Kenya, Slovenia, UK, and Uruguay, among many other countries. He also is an award-winning poet, having published fourteen books of original poetry and poetry in translation. His work has been translated into multiple languages, including Hindi, Italian, Serbian, Slovenian, Spanish, and Vietnamese, and he is a highly sought speaker across the globe. After leading poetry workshops for three years in the most restrictive maximum-security detention center in the US for undocumented, unaccompanied youth, he edited and translated the bilingual poetry anthology *Dreaming America: Voices of Undocumented Youth in Maximum-Security Detention* (Settlement House, 2017), with the proceeds from its sale going to a legal defense fund for incarcerated, undocumented youth. Of further note, the poetry in *Dreaming America* has been turned into original music by two different, celebrated composers, and it has been turned into two different plays.

Email: michelsons@wlu.edu

Postal Address: Washington and Lee University. Romance Languages Department

204 W. Washington St. Lexington, VA 24450.

Contribution: "Looking for Luz."

Abigail Nunez-Saenz is the daughter of two Mexican immigrants. She was born and raised in the Rio Grande Valley where she has been able to explore her Mexican heritage all while figuring out what it means to be Estadounidense. She is a graduate of the University of Texas Rio Grande Valley where she obtained a Bachelor of Science in Psychology and a Master of Education in Special Education. Throughout her undergraduate career, she presented research in regional, state, and national conferences involving populations such as DACA, immigrants and refugees, and people with developmental disabilities. She is currently pursuing a certification in Applied Behavior Analysis.

Email: abigailnzs96@gmail.com

Postal Address: 411 Agua Viva Ln., Brownsville, TX., 78521

Contribution: With Briones and al, "Buscando un destino."

Paola Quijano obtained her bachelor's degree in psychological science at the University of Texas Rio Grande Valley in 2017. As an undergraduate Ms. Quijano spent her time researching the resiliency among marginalized communities, this led her to volunteer at the Humanitarian Respite Center located in South Texas. Ms. Quijano developed a passion for advocating on behalf of others and decided to continue her studies. In 2019 Ms. Quijano graduated with a Master of Science in Clinical Rehabilitation Counseling, she is currently living in Austin, TX where she works as a therapist for children with special needs. As a first-generation Mexican American Ms. Quijano takes pride in representing Latinx heritage through her work.

Email: paola.mirandaquijano@gmail.com

Postal Address: 5708 W Parmer Ln Apt 13106 Austin, TX 78727

Contribution: With Briones and al, "Buscando un destino."

Jaime Retamales, originally from Chile, is a Visiting Assistant Professor of Spanish at Lamar University in Beaumont, TX. Dr. Retamales field of research is Latin-American Literature, especially Chilean literature. Dr. Retamales focus is exile literature, indigenous, and LGBT. Dr. Retamales has presented in several conferences in the United States. He has published articles in several American journals. He edits papers for *Lamar Journal of Humanities*. Dr. Retamales has a column in the Chilean Newspaper *El Morrocotudo* where he publishes his articles.

Email: jretamales@gmail.com

Postal Address: 2163 Tree LN, Kingwood, TX 77339

Contribution: "Jeremías"

Juan Ríos Vega is an assistant professor in the Department of Education, Counseling, and Leadership at Bradley University. As a critical race and LatCrit scholar, Dr. Ríos Vega analyzes how social identities intersect different layers of oppression, shaping Latinx communities in schools in the United States. He also documents the experiences of LGBTIQ+ individuals in Panama, his homeland. His research studies have been presented at local and international conferences. Dr. Ríos Vega is the author of *Counter storytelling narratives of Latino teenage boys: From "vergüenza" to "échale ganas,"* (Peter Lang Publishing, 2015), *Historias desde el sexilio,* (Impresora Pacífico, 2018), and *High school Latinx counternarratives: Experiences in School and Post-graduation,* (Peter Lang Publishing, 2020), and his first bilingual children's book *Carlos, The Fairy Boy/ Carlos, El Niño Hada* (Reflection Press, 2020).

Email: jariosvega@gmail.com, jriosvega@bradley.edu

Postal Address: 1015 North Institute Place, Peoria, IL, 61606

Contribution: "An ESL Classroom as a Healing Space."

Andy Torres is a Clinical Psychology Masters student at The University of Texas Rio Grande Valley (UTRGV) and the Graduate Research Assistant at the Multicultural Clinical Lab and BeChilD Lab. He is a 1st generation, Latinx, English-as-Second-Language college student aiming to make significant contributions in the mental health field. Andy intends to become an LPC, a BCBA, and a Licensed Psychologist. He aspires to work as a clinical neuro-rehabilitation psychologist upon a Ph.D./post-doc completion. He also dreams to make significant research and clinical impacts on the Latinx community and make mental health / ABA services more readily available to the underserved communities. When he is not working on manuscripts & research projects, attending classes, or working with children/adults with NDDs, Andy loves to take nature photography, write poetry, and to take mini (and big) trips with his loved ones.

Email: andytorres632@gmail.com, andy.torres01@utrgv.edu

Postal Address: 419 Arron St. Donna, Texas. 78537.

Contribution: With Briones and al, "Buscando un destino."

Francisco J. Villegas is an Assistant Professor of Sociology in the Department of Anthropology and Sociology at Kalamazoo College. His research focuses on the intersection of race and immigration status, particularly how they are employed to maintain borders to membership and the ways migrants mobilize to resist these exclusions. He has co-edited two books: *Seeds of Hope: Creating a Future in the Shadows* and *Critical Schooling: Transformative Theory and Practice* and published various academic journal articles and book chapters.

Email: francisco.villegas@kzoo.edu

Postal Address: 1200 Academy Dr. Kalamazoo, MI 49006

Contribution: With P. Villegas, "Reflection on schooling experiences as undocumented migrants in the U.S"

Paloma E. Villegas is an interdisciplinary artist and assistant professor of sociology at California State University San Bernardino. Her research examines the production of migrant illegalization Mexico, the U.S. and Canada and its intersections with borders, race, gender, class, and nation-building. She is the author of *North of El Norte: Illegalized Mexican Migrants in Canada* (forthcoming, University of British Columbia Press).

Email: pvillegas24@gmail.com

Postal Address: 5500 University Parkway San Bernardino, CA, 92407 USA

Contribution: Los Niños Florero with F. Villegas, "Reflection on schooling experiences as undocumented migrants in the U.S"

Amanda Venta, Ph.D. is an Associate Professor in the Department of Psychology at the University of Houston. Her research focuses on attachment between parents and children and how the quality of these attachments relates to mental health and well-being at biological and behavioral levels. Her interest in attachment disruptions spurred her focus on Central American immigration, a context in which families are often separated for long periods of time. She is a first generation American herself and has provided psychological services to unaccompanied immigrant minors in the custody of the Office of Refugee Resettlement since 2012, including graduate students in that experience since 2015. Her research has been funded by the National Institute of Mental Health, the National Institute of Minority Health and Health Disparities, and the American Psychological Foundation. She has authored or co-authored three books, 16 chapters, and more than 80 manuscripts. Notable among these contributions are an edited volume textbook entitled *Developmental Psychopathology* for students of psychology and articles published in the *Journal of the American Academy of Child and Adolescent Psychiatry*, the *Journal of Clinical Child and Adolescent Psychology*, *Psychological Assessment*, and *Attachment and Human Development*.

Email: aventa@uh.edu

Postal Address: The University of Houston, Health 1, 4849 Calhoun Road, Room 373, Houston, TX 77204-6022

Contribution: With Montse Feu "Introduction: Serving Refugee Children and their Families."

Translators

Dr. Mercedes Fernández Asenjo is a lecturer of Spanish at Binghamton University SUNY. Dr.

Fernández-Asenjo has a Ph.D. in US Hispanic Literature from the University of Houston and a certificate in Women's and Gender Studies from that same institution. Her research focuses on the Dominican Republic, specifically on the development of the feminist movement in that country and how women involved in it established a network of international relations with other Latin American countries and the US. Dr. Fernández Asenjo was recipient of a NEH Fellowship to attend the Summer Institute "Women's Suffrage in the Americas" in Carthage College (2018). She has presented her research on national and international academic conferences and has published articles and a book chapter in peer-reviewed journals and academic presses in the United States and the Dominican Republic. She is now working on an article about Dominican fin-de-siècle author Virginia Elena Ortea and her association to Hostos' ideas on women and society.

Email: fernandm@binghamton.edu

Postal Address: 110 East 40th st suite 301, 10016 New York NY

Translation: "Un viaje indocumentado en busca de un corazón."

Montse Feu is an associate professor of Hispanic Studies at Sam Houston State University. She recovers the literary history of the Spanish Civil War exile in the United States, U.S., Hispanic periodicals, and migration literature at large. She migrated to the USA in 2005 and is a first-generation scholar. She is the author of *Correspondencia personal y política de un anarcosindicalista exiliado: Jesús González Malo (1943–1965)* (Universidad de Cantabria, 2016) and *Fighting Fascist Spain,* (University of Illinois Press, 2020), She is co-editor of *Writing Revolution: Hispanic Anarchism in the United States* (University of Illinois Press, 2019). She is board member for the Recovering the U. S. Hispanic Literary Heritage and for the Research Society for American Periodicals.

Email: mmf017@shsu.edu

Address: 7 Moonseed Place. The Woodlands. Texas 77381, USA.

Translations:

"Una reflexión sobre su propia escolarización como migrantes indocumentados en los EE. UU."

"El aula de inglés como segunda lengua: un lugar de sanación,"

Betsy E. Galicia was born and raised in Houston, Texas to Mexican parents. She graduated from the University of Houston with a Bachelor's in Science degree in Psychology and a minor in Biology. In 2016, she graduated from

John Jay College of Criminal Justice in New York, primarily working with ethnic minority and immigrant justice-involved youth. Since 2017, she has been working towards earning her doctoral degree at Sam Houston State University in clinical psychology. Her work primarily focuses on immigrant youth, trauma, protective and risk factors in developing psychopathology, and diversity issues.

Email: bgalicia@shsu.edu

Postal Address: 1087 Verde Trails Dr. Houston TX 77073

Translation: "Creciendo Muy Rápido."

Wendy Herrera Fernandez is a Spanish teacher and department chair in Nimitz Ninth grade. Ms. Herrera focuses on teaching vocabulary and grammar in a meaningful context and emphasizes the importance of learning the cultural aspects of the language. She seeks to increase student's awareness, which in turn strengthens student's motivation and attitude towards learning. Ms. Herrera is an alumna from Sam Houston State University. With a bachelor's degree in criminal justice and a Master of Arts in Spanish, her education has allowed her to understand individuality from an educational and criminological perspective. One of the areas she investigates is the impact of translations and interpretations (English-Spanish, Spanish-English) in the criminal justice system. After all, scholars "by their very nature, love puzzles [,] they love to figure out complex relationships and discover how processes work" (Wright & Boisvert 2009), and that's what research provides to individuals, the opportunity to create new insights on areas that have never been looked at before.

Email: herrerawendy438@gmail.com, wendy.herrera21@yahoo.com

Postal Address: 143 Hollyvale Dr. Houston, TX 77060

Translations: "Silencio," "Camila," "Buscando a Luz."

Tara Marshall is a SHSU graduate with a B.A. in Spanish and a minor in Mass Communications. She has received several honors including being a Who's Who Among Students in American Universities and Colleges Award Recipient and graduating Suma Cum Lade. She has also published several pieces for the Houstonian Newspaper. She plans on continuing her studies in language and teaching foreign languages abroad. She has been working on a comic set to release this year on Webtoons Discover called Darling, Darling: Superhero Stories.

Email: tara_marshall@sbchlobal.net

Postal Address: 645 Topaz Ln, Leander, TX 78641

Translation: "Jeremías"

Blanca Tovar (Blanca Patricia Tovar Frias) is from México. She studied the Bachelor and master's degree in Pedagogy at Universidad Nacional Autónoma de México. Her Master's Thesis "Resistencia Educativa hacia el Proyecto Institucional de Secundaria: Una mirada de los estudiantes de la Secundaria Técnica N° 24" has been published by Editorial Académica Española. In 2017, she graduated from the Master of Arts in Spanish, Sam Houston State University. During summer 2017, spring 2018, and summer 2018, Blanca was a Research Assistant in the project "Spanish Civil War Exile in the United States and US Latinx Literature: Exiles, Migrants and Refugees", led by Dr. Montse Feu, Associate Professor of Hispanic Studies at Sam Houston State University. In 2018, she worked as Spanish Adjunct of Faculty in Continuing Education at Montgomery Lone Star College, Texas. In 2019, Blanca worked a High School Spanish Teacher for a short time at Houston, Texas. Currently she is not working in the education field.

Email: blanca.tovar@yahoo.com

Postal Address:2200 Montgomery Park Blvd. #501. Conroe, TX.,77304

Translation: "El amor de extraños."

Printed in the USA
CPSIA information can be obtained
at www.ICGtesting.com
LVHW010801100624
782767LV00004B/298

9 781433 179495